Samuel J. Tibbitts • Allen J. Manzano

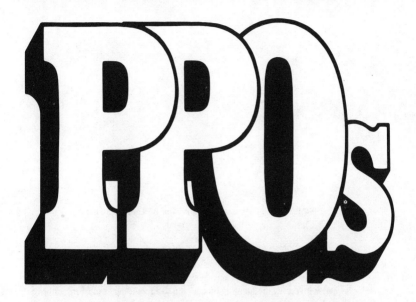

PREFERRED PROVIDER ORGANIZATIONS
•AN EXECUTIVE'S GUIDE•

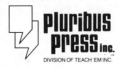

pluribus
press inc.
DIVISION OF TEACH 'EM INC.

Library of Congress Catalog Card Number:
83-62497

International Standard Book Number:
0-931028-40-X

Pluribus Press, Inc., Division of Teach'em, Inc.
160 East Illinois Street
Chicago, Illinois 60611

Printed in the United States of America

Acknowledgments

The authors gratefully acknowledge the invaluable assistance of Tyler Artz, Russell Coile, Nicholas Moss and, with special commendation, Inez Kimi Mann.

Chapter drafts in progress were reviewed by Lois Green; Debbie Harrison; Terry Hartshorn; Allan Hoops; Catherine A. Kay, Esquire, of Konowiecki, Keast & Brown; and Edith Strevey.

James E. Ludlam, Esquire, of Musick, Peeler & Garrett, contributed incisive comments and made a substantial contribution to the legal issues chapter by sharing his thoughts on malpractice.

Anne Dillibe and Dennis Strum were instrumental in expediting bibliographic research and review.

To these individuals—our friends and colleagues—our thanks and sincere appreciation.

October 1983

Contents

Exhibits

CHAPTER ONE

The PPO—What It Is

Defining a PPO is like slicing batter, for the PPO cake has yet to be baked.

The term Preferred Provider Organization (PPO) is in the process of evolution: it is an open and permissive phrase, one without rigid criteria that excludes any player. Yesterday, you never heard of a PPO; today, you are being invited to join one. Yesterday, you were organizing health care and financing a delivery scheme; today, you discover that you are a PPO.

The most formal attempt at defining a PPO may be found in the AHA publication, "Defining Our Own Future; An American Hospital Association Glossary."[1] In this publication, the AHA defines the PPO as follows:

> A payment arrangement where insurers contract with hospitals or physicians on a fee-for-services basis to provide health care services. Subscribers can select any provider for care but they are given economic or other incentives to use these designated hospitals or physicians.

The AHA definition, while not inaccurate, is probably too narrow in scope: it is not necessarily true that the payment arrangement would be on a fee-for-service basis. Nor is it necessarily true that the program would involve only hospitals or physicians.

The generally acknowledged source of the term Preferred Provider Organization is Linda Ellwein of Interstudy, the Minneapolis-based health think tank, who called the emerging structures "Preferred Provider Organizations."[2]

This term itself grew out of Ellwein's awareness of a new kind of entity under the more general grouping of Alternate Delivery Systems, in which Interstudy has had a continuing interest. Ellwein's definition was guided by a set of observed common characteristics. These were:

- Provider panel with a limited number of "preferred" physicians and hospitals.

- Negotiated fee schedule (frequently considered a discount).

- Utilization or claims review and some form of control mechanism for utilization and costs.

- Consumers not "locked in" with additional benefits created to encourage use of PPO providers.
- Rapid turnaround on provider claims.

Ellwein's list of characteristics has probably been exceeded by PPOs that have evolved beyond these limits in such areas as range of providers, financial arrangements and systems requirements.

Toward a Working Definition

Because of the evolutionary nature of the term, we offer the following as a working definition:

> A *Preferred Provider Organization* is a health financing and delivery arrangement in which a group of health care providers offers its services on a predetermined financial basis to health care purchasers under terms which encourage selection of the providers as the source of service to sponsored individuals.

Let's review that definition on a phrase-by-phrase basis.

"A health financing and delivery structure"

The PPO is a new variation on the continuing evolution of health delivery and financing structures. An outgrowth of the existing fee-for-service and insurance (for which also read "Indemnity Plan") programs, the PPO owes a particular debt to the concept of dual choice insurance, where sponsored individuals select from options that involve them in greater or lesser financial risk keyed to the range of services and degree of cost sharing. PPOs also share some of the elements of health maintenance organizations (HMOs), particularly in unifying providers under some kind of organizational structure. PPOs parallel HMOs in their design, using private physician panels or the Independent Practitioner Association (IPA) model. It can be argued that the earliest

conceptual models for the PPO were Blue Cross and Blue
Shield, both of which—in their beginnings—represented some
limitations on freedom of choice. As these plans grew, however,
they lost the element of selectivity. Deriving as they do from
these sources, PPOs must include health delivery and financing
under some kind of organizational plan. A major distinction
must be noted in that providers do not, in a PPO, assume an
insurance risk. The providers do, however, participate in arrangements which may involve them in substantial business
risks.

"A group of health care providers offering their services"

In *every* PPO, there must be a group of providers with the capacity to offer a reasonable range of services to targeted groups.
The provider grouping typically includes hospitals and physicians, but a PPO's providers group is, if nothing else, flexible.
It can and, over time, probably would incorporate whatever mix
of providers might fit a particular group's service expectations.
Some of the other likely service participants are dentists, podiatrists, home health agencies, long-term care facilities, pharma-
cies and surgi-centers. However, the initial PPO associations are
primarily focused on hospitals and physicians. This is because
together they represent the greatest proportion of the insured
health care dollar. They are also mutually dependent in offering
their respective services and have established organizational
linkages. Hospitals, in particular, also have the resources and
structures required to establish and participate in such new entities.

"On a predetermined financial basis"

The PPO invariably establishes a financial arrangement on a
contractual basis in advance of service delivery. The financial
arrangement is designed primarily to offer cost advantages to the
purchaser of service and business volume (or preservation of
market share) to the provider of service. The arrangement is

commonly the result of negotiation, of offer and counter offer, with the payor and provider reaching accommodation based upon their perceptions of presumed and reasonable advantage. The nature and degree of negotiation is conditioned by specific and highly localized marketing phenomena such as competition, capacity, demand and cost, as well as legal requirements. In California, however, negotiation has been limited, with many providers merely given the choice of accepting or rejecting *in toto* the offered contractual terms.

"To health care purchasers"

It takes a secure source of service payment to create an operational PPO. The purchaser, however, exists in many guises. The most likely and, often, the most preferred by the provider is an insurer with the ability to design and offer insurance programs to a large number of groups in a given market. However, a contracted purchaser could be a self-insured group, a multi-employer trust fund, a union trust fund, an insurance brokerage house, an indemnity payer or a government agency.

"Under terms which encourage selection of providers as the source of service by a sponsored individual"

Here is the crux of the matter: *The PPO is meaningless unless it is effective in delivering patients to the organization's providers.* The aim is, however, preserving a provider's bottom line, not necessarily generating greater volume but ensuring the right patient mix.

Without affecting the choice of provider incentives, the program is merely a discount scheme. These incentives are typically financial in nature and involve a cost penalty to a user of service who goes outside the system's parameters. By the same token, a program must offer sufficient numbers of providers with acceptable geographic distribution for service access. These conditions ensure access to service without queuing or excessive travel to a delivery site and are crucial to a successful PPO. A program would fail to meet our definition if the user of service did not have a real choice but was required to use the provider network, as would be the case in an exclusive provider organization.

We will discuss the options and choices available within our definition in much of the rest of this book. In general, we expect that the PPOs that will ultimately emerge will share at least these general characteristics—characteristics which are, in effect, governed by the key adjective "preferred."

Driving Forces

The health care system has been in continuing turmoil over the last two decades, coping with rapid changes in the social and economic environment and with the products of technological and organizational development. The darling of Wall Street, and one of the real juggernauts of the American service economy, health care is a fluid and expanding industry. New conditions of enormous consequence are created by the stroke of a government pen and, almost as quickly, multiple and effective responses emerge to meet them. The PPO, in effect, is only one of the series of the many products emerging from this process of change and our willingness to experiment and to institutionalize such experiments often without clear evidence that they will, in fact, work.

And PPOs are an exploding phenomenon. If California is a bellwether as it often is, then there can be every expectation of an initial, very rapid national growth in the PPO field, particuarly in terms of organization and development. In California, information from the Department of Corporations indicates that some 150 PPOs are now in the process of organization. Of course, the problem here again is that one needs only to declare oneself a PPO, since there is as yet no legal definition. It is probably reasonable to expect a stressful and rigorous weeding out of these organizations, as poorly designed entities without staying power begin to fall by the wayside.

But, the questions remain: why are PPOs developing; what conditions are stimulating this rapid development? Inflationary pressures. Recession. Increased competition. These have been real for all health care sectors. The trends that influence life in general in the United States have had significant impact upon insurers, consumers of health care services, employer groups and providers of services.

There can be no real understanding of the PPO phenomenon without a basic understanding of the insurance industry's perspective with respect to health care costs. The insurance industry has a protracted history of underwriting health insurance losses. These losses were generally subsidized through other lines of insurance and, in part, by cash flow underwriting. That trend continues: in 1979, after deduction of operating expenses, private health insurers lost $1.4 billion; in 1978, the loss underwritten was $1.5 billion.[3]

The period 1950–1979 saw a 2,900 per cent increase per capita in insurance premium expenses.[4] That per capita cost continues to rise: renewal rate increases for group medical insurance in 1982, it has been reported, will be higher than the 30 per cent reported by major health insurers in 1981.[5] Exacerbating the problems, and contributing to the magnitude of the cost problem, is the practice of cost shifting: the private sector will subsidize the public sector by about $5.8 billion in 1982 (vs. $4.8 billion in 1981).[6]

Several other trends are noteworthy:

● Despite the rise in premium rates, the insurance benefit structure has not kept pace with hospital and physician expenditures.

● The traditional, private health insurer faces the prospect of diminished market share. There has been a steady rise toward self-funding by employers. It is now estimated that one-third of all labor-management plans are self-insured. As

of 1980, state governments show a similar trend of self-insurance for their employees. (See exhibit 1.1)
- New health insurance policy plans show an apparent shift away from full contributions by the employer, with consequent cost sharing by the employee.

(Those interested in a more comprehensive and authoritative discussion of private health insurance are referred to "Private Health Insurance Plans in 1978 and 1979: A Major Review of Coverage, Enrollment and Financial Experience," by Marjorie Smith Carroll and Ross H. Arnett III, in the *Health Care Financing Review,* September 1981.)

The consumer of health care is directly impacted by these trends. During the period 1950–1979, the per capita premium rose from $8.57 to $254.34. The percentage of personal income devoted to health insurance rose from 0.6 per cent to 3.4 per cent. (See exhibit 1.2)

Even more important to the consumer, health insurance has begun to pay a diminished proportion of expenditures. In 1979, private health insurance paid 44.7 per cent of the $112.2 billion consumers spent on personal health care. Personal health care cost—noncovered or partially covered—was 55.3 per cent, direct and out-of-pocket. In 1978, by contrast, private health insurance covered 45.4 per cent of expenditures, the consumer, 54.6 per cent. As more personal resources are committed to health care, the consumer obviously has less to devote to other purchases.

As exhibit 1.3 makes clear, the total expenditures paid for by private health insurance rose from 12.2 per cent in 1950 and peaked at 45.4 per cent in 1978. A slight downtrend has been apparent for every year after 1976, in the percentage of costs covered for hospital and physician services.

Because employers pay approximately 26 per cent of total health care costs (approximately $75 billion), the proliferation of business coalitions seeking to contain medical care costs and utilization was to be expected, given the sharp rise in the cost of

Exhibit 1.1
Percentage of Health Insurance Business

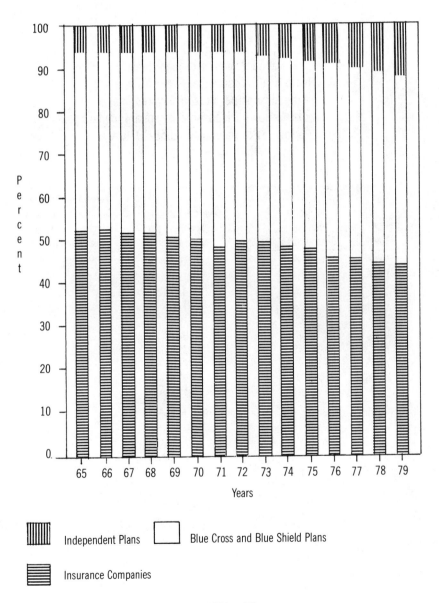

Exhibit 1.2
Per Capita Premium Expenditures for
Private Health Insurance, Average Premium
Expenditures per Person Covered, and
Percentage of National Disposable Personal Income Spent
for Health Insurance, 1950-1979

Year	Per Capita Premium Expenditures	Average Premium Expenditure per Person Covered	Percent of National Disposable Personal Income Spent for Health Insurance
1950	$ 8.57	$ 16.85	0.6
1955	19.33	29.25	1.1
1960	32.79	44.26	1.7
1965	51.80	72.29	2.1
1970	84.09	110.69	2.5
1975	152.73	198.01	3.0
1976	178.49	232.42	3.2
1977	206.93	264.98	3.4
1978	228.56	293.91	3.4
1979	254.34	327.06	3.4

Health Care Financing Review, September 1981, p. 84.

Exhibit 1.3
Percentage of Expenditures Paid by Insurance

Year	Total	Hospital Care	Physicians' Services	Prescribed Drugs (Out-of-Hospital)	Dental Care	Other Types of Care
1950	12.2	37.1	12.0	1	1	1
1960	27.8	64.7	30.0	1	1	5.0
1965	32.1	70.9	34.0	2.6	1.5	3.1
1966	31.9	70.9	33.9	2.9	1.8	3.5
1967	33.7	77.2	36.8	3.6	2.3	5.0
1968	34.7	77.2	39.3	3.0	2.4	4.3
1969	35.9	77.5	40.5	3.3	3.0	5.2
1970	37.5	78.2	42.9	4.1	5.4	4.9
1971	38.4	79.6	42.6	4.7	5.9	5.2
1972	38.1	75.8	45.0	4.9	6.2	5.3
1973	38.1	73.8	45.5	5.5	7.0	5.8
1974	40.2	76.2	49.4	6.1	8.1	6.1
1975	43.6	81.3	50.9	6.8	13.0	5.6
1976	45.2	81.3	52.7	8.0	17.7	5.6
1977	45.1	79.2	52.3	8.7	18.8	6.0
1978	45.4	80.4	50.7	9.2	20.4	6.1
1979	44.7	79.1	48.9	9.9	22.3	5.9

Source: National Health Accounts, Division of National Cost Estimates, Office of Financial and Actuarial Analysis, HCFA.
[1]Data are not available.
Health Care Financing Review, September 1981, p. 85.

benefit plans.[7] It has been estimated that 25 per cent of the $540 billion spent for employee benefits goes to fund health care. This represents, to the employer, approximately $1,000/employee.[8] (*Modern Healthcare,* 83/01, p. 62, attributed to R. Kahn and J. J. May).

One tactic to reduce medical costs to business has been the redesign of medical benefits plans. A recent survey found that approximately 20 per cent of the responding firms increased employees' share of costs through raising individual, family or combined deductibles.[9] Other firms have reduced limits on payment of hospital benefits.

If the problem has been severe for the private sector, it is the public sector that has experienced the sharpest spiral of health care program costs. Since the enactment of the Medicare and Medicaid programs in the mid-1960s, federal government outlays for health care have risen from $4.7 billion in 1957 to $46.6 billion in fiscal year 1982 for Medicare. The funds committed to Medicaid have risen from $1.5 billion in 1957 to $17.4 billion in fiscal year 1982. By one projection, *total* federal outlays for health care are expected to increase from $74 billion in fiscal year 1982 to $144 billion in fiscal year 1988.[10]

Health care represented only 4.4 per cent of the gross national product (GNP) in 1950. It expanded to 9.8 per cent of GNP in 1981 and 10.5 per cent in 1982. The past federal philosophy of open access to health care services, since modified by the Reagan administration, was reflected in the ballooning amounts committed to health care funding. That philosophy substantially increased demand and stimulated the use of hospital care through expansion of third-party coverage, principally through the Medicare and Medicaid programs.

Current projections by Mark S. Freeland and Carol Ellen Schendler, printed in *Health Care Financing Review,* Winter 1981, foresee total national health expenditures rising to $462.2 billion in 1985 and $821 billion in 1990. "This growth," they note, "continues the historical trend in which health spending has doubled every six years."[11] Exhibit 1.4 illustrates their point.

Freeland and Schendler's forecast also predicts that the sources of funds to finance health expenditures have and will continue to shift over time. By 1990, the federal government is seen as the source of 32 per cent of all health care payments, while private funds will account for 54 per cent, and local funds for 14 per cent. (See exhibit 1.5)

It has been one of the accepted shibboleths of our age that providers (principally hospitals) have been in large part responsible for the health care cost spiral. More thoughtful analysts have noted that federal policy and payment mechanisms have played a critical role in the direction of health care expenditure growth. Recent studies have shown, too, that fiscal stress in hospitals is clearly not the result of mismanagement, inefficiency or under use. The patient and service mix (e.g., high volumes of charity and Medicaid patients and a high bad debt load) have been demonstrated to have more to do with fiscal stress than hospital operations. The study by Hadley, Feder and Mullner notes:[12]

> . . . the problem of hospital financial distress becomes obvious—
> a hospital cannot provide service without compensation and
> remain financially viable. To a large extent, then, the hospital
> problem of financial stress overlaps the social problem of financ-
> ing health care for the poor. If people without resources are to
> receive care, somebody else has to pay.

The problem of payment for uncompensated care is addressed only peripherally by the PPO. It can be argued that seeking competitive advantage for the provider by concentrating on increasing the private pay patient base strengthens the fiscal position of any provider, thereby allowing the provider to remain financially viable and provide some modicum of service to the poor.

While it is a given that costs have escalated, better general

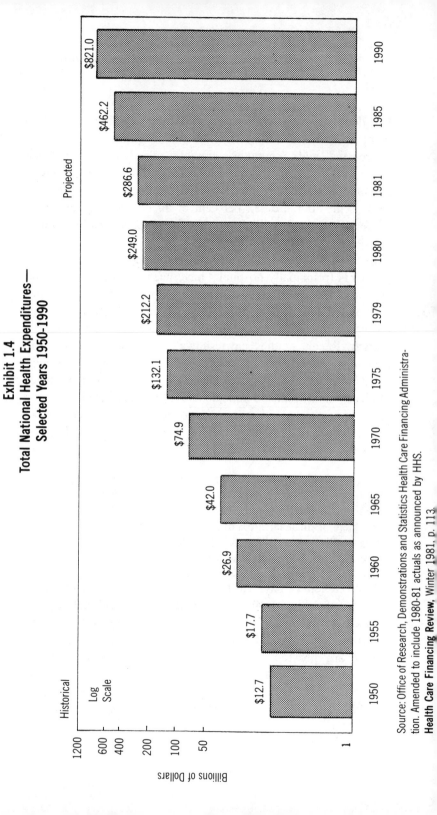

Exhibit 1.4
Total National Health Expenditures—
Selected Years 1950-1990

Source: Office of Research, Demonstrations and Statistics Health Care Financing Administration. Amended to include 1980-81 actuals as announced by HHS. **Health Care Financing Review**, Winter 1981, p. 113.

Exhibit 1.5
Percent Distribution of Total National Health Expenditures by Source of Funds for Selected Years, 1950-1979

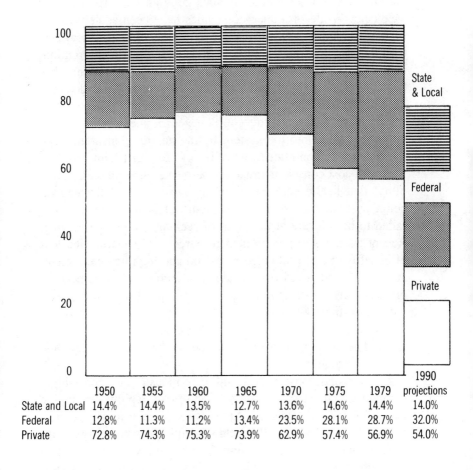

	1950	1955	1960	1965	1970	1975	1979	1990 projections
State and Local	14.4%	14.4%	13.5%	12.7%	13.6%	14.6%	14.4%	14.0%
Federal	12.8%	11.3%	11.2%	13.4%	23.5%	28.1%	28.7%	32.0%
Private	72.8%	74.3%	75.3%	73.9%	62.9%	57.4%	56.9%	54.0%

Health Care Financing Review, Winter 1981, p. 114 (amended).

understanding of the cost problem is freeing health care providers from simplistic accusatory charges of fiscal irresponsibility. These concerns have also gone beyond the legislative and regulatory coping of governments unwilling or unable to pay for the full cost consequences of such programs as Medicare or Medicaid. While insurance companies have been acutely aware of the problems of health care costs, particularly as it affects their bottom line and ability to remain within their premium income, it is only lately that the general business community has begun to focus on the health care cost problem and to understand its complexity. There is now a general acknowledgement that the problem is largely the consequence of the incentives that have been built into the system by the nature of insurance and the financially conditioned behavior of users of health care.

Health cost consciousness does permeate our economic sensibility: that health care cost is excessive is part of the general belief system. Nevertheless, the issue of health care cost has failed to be relevant at the point of seeking health care service. Recent cutbacks in government resources and benefits, the loss of benefits due to prolonged recession and high unemployment, and private sector efforts to scale back employee health benefits programs are creating an awareness of costs at the point of service utilization. Ultimately, this growing emphasis on costs at the point of utilization will impel the emergence of new structures. The development of PPOs ideally matches this new and growing incentive system.

Market conditions in the health care industry are increasingly competitive, most significantly because of a rapidly developing excess of delivery capacity. An early example of a major capacity problem has been in the field of dentistry, where large numbers of practitioners have come into the market precisely at a time when demand for service has flattened. A similar pattern is developing in medicine, where doctors are emerging from the training pipeline at rates in excess of replacement and market growth requirements. Lastly, hospitals, with their huge investments in fixed plants, and offering services with limited flexibility and costly conversion, are finding that enforced planning has not given them market monopoly. They have found, too, that the growth of alternative free-standing delivery structures is intensifying competition. In effect, hospitals are seeing that the fluidity of the delivery system no longer assures universal survival.

PPOs, in fact, are probably not viable in areas where competition does not threaten existing market shares of present providers and where there is little prospect of any competition emerging in the near to mid term. Eagerness to organize or participate in PPOs is thus directly proportional to the degree to which an area's providers perceive the new competitive market and feel themselves threatened in their market share by new delivery components.

Heretofore, government intervention has inhibited effective competition and minimized the need for such structures as PPOs. Government has been particularly anti-competition in its attempt to regulate facilities development and in its use of cost-based reimbursement in the financing of Medicare and Medicaid since these programs were established in 1965.

A payment program based on cost (no matter how rigidly defined) motivates providers to develop reimbursement maximization strategies rather than competitive strategies. As government shifts to either bidding arrangements or fixed price schedules, provider concerns will focus on price competition and product selection. The prototype for a bidding arrangement already exists in California, where the Medicaid program has been bid out of hospitals on a negotiated price basis and where the state expects to enter into similar arrangements with other providers. The shift to fixed price schedules is already underway in Medicare, where payment by admission and the development of a case mix payment methodology is having a powerful effect on hospital financing, organization and management. The cost reimbursement system essentially provides a safety net to the provider. A fixed price system eliminates that margin of safety. The inefficient provider can no longer rely upon having costs covered and must strictly monitor cost efficiency for survival. The loss of a government purchaser for all or for certain services and/or the inability to recoup the costs of service to government sponsored patients will clearly signal hospitals that they must review product line and market position in regard to other sources of payment. In such an environment, the patient mix becomes crucially important. The PPO is an ideal vehicle by which to provide a hospital with access to such new markets without disturbing its internal organizational structure and with limited adjustments to its service, price, and contractual arrangements.

Probably the most significant change in the federal government's approach to health care financing is its emphasis on financial incentive, particularly in that it is validating and encouraging profit and favorable operating margins rather than discouraging them. Another crucial development has been the Reagan Administration's commitment to changing the financial arrangements for health care in the private sector as well. *The Tax Equity and Fiscal Responsibility Act of 1983, which began to restrict the deductibility of health care costs to the individual and employers, is only the beginning of a general move to provide dollar incentives to the American consumer to buy and use health care services prudently.*

While there are many potential organizational responses to these new incentives and changes in the health care environment, preferred provider organizations can help hospitals and other providers focus on aggressive competition and marketing as the ways to survive and prosper.

Notes

1. Defining Our Own Future: An American Hospital Association Glossary. American Hospital Association. January 1983.

2. Ellwein, Linda. Interstudy Internal Memo, February 1981.
3. Carroll, Marjorie Smith and Arnett, Ross H. III. Private Health Insurance Plans in 1978 and 1979: A Review of Coverage, Enrollment, and Financial Experience. *Health Care Financing Review.* (3)1:55, September 1981.
4. Ibid., p. 84.
5. Rundle, Rhonda L. No Relief From Rate Hikes; Health Plan Insurers Factor In Runaway Costs. *Business Insurance.* (16)22:1. May 31, 1982.
6. Ibid.
7. Glueck, David L. Trends in Health Care Costs. *Pension World.* (18)11:49–50. November 1982.
8. Coalitions Hungry for Hospital Data. *Modern Healthcare.* (13)1:-62. January 1983.
9. *Op. Cit.,* p. 50.
10. Statement of the American Hospital Association, before the Senate Committee on Labor and Human Resources on Health Care Cost, May 25, 1983.
11. Freedland, Mark S. and Schendler, Carol Ellen. National Health Expenditures: Short-Term Outlook and Long-Term Projections. *Health Care Financing Review.* (2)3:111. Winter 1981.
12. Hadley, Jack; Feder, Judith; and Mullner, Ross. "Care for the Poor and Hospitals Financial Status: Results of a Survey of Hospitals in Large Cities." Draft Report, undated. p. 27.

CHAPTER TWO
Feasibility Analysis

The principal purpose of the feasibility analysis is to determine if indeed a market exists for a PPO.

This evaluation entails a market analysis, organizational assessment, consideration of alternative PPO designs and the development of an implementation plan. The market assessment highlights the broad external pressures impacting the hospital industry, as well as local and regional conditions influencing the health care marketplace.

Through the evaluation of the external environment, a thorough assessment can be made of the business community's concern for cost containment and industry's organization of coalitions or other measures to address the cost containment issue. To date, coalitions have taken little action to aggressively structure or develop PPOs. However, industry's specific actions to contain costs on a national, as well as local, basis should be considered in the analysis. The impact of legislation and proposed legislation should be considered, as this too will influence the marketplace for the PPO delivery system. Also, the experience of providers or other groups in developing and organizing PPOs should be assessed to guide the development of a well conceived, appropriately designed program.

This type of assessment provides a general understanding of forces and factors influencing PPO development. It also provides a better perspective as to the opportunities available in the development of preferred provider organizations.

While the foregoing factors yield a reasonably broad-based external evaluation, a review of the local market must also be conducted. This provides specific information regarding market size, population and demographics, profile of major purchasers of health care (insurance companies, self-insured employers and trusts) and current purchase patterns. The review should entail analysis of the following:

- Industry Profile:

  - Number and size of employers—including presence of corporate headquarters, mid to large size companies

- Insurance arrangements, especially self-insured companies
- Dominant brokers and consultants
- HMOs, PPOs or other alternative delivery mechanisms offered and penetration levels
- Prevailing benefit structures, especially the prevalence of plans compatible with a dual option plan

● Population/Demographics:

- Past and present by location, age, and sex
- Future projections by location, age, and sex
- Utilization patterns and rates
- Employment patterns and rates

● Provider Profile:

- Current industry usage and buyers
- Past and present market share
- Primary and referral service area
- Changes over time
- Number and type of physicians, as well as prevalence of group practice arrangements

● Competition Profile:

- Market share and penetration levels
- Current industry relationships and/or anticipation in alternative delivery systems
- Financial performance and viability
- Perceived strengths and weaknesses

In addition to the evaluation of the market structure itself, there should also be an understanding of behavior and attitudes in the marketplace. This is extremely beneficial in obtaining a subtle, or qualitative, perspective of the market. Areas of focus include the following:

● Industry Behavior:

- Coalition actions and plans

- Plans for PPO contracts

- Attitudes toward cost-containment and PPOs

- Opinions of participating hospitals and competing institutions

- Actions and plans regarding health insurance arrangements

- Opinions of HMOs and alternative delivery systems

● Physician Behavior:

- Reactions and opinions of industry's activities

- Attitudes toward private utilization review, discounts, and PPOs

- Attitudes toward HMOs

- Attitudes toward participating hospitals

● Insurance Behavior:

- Plans for PPOs

- Attitudes toward PPOs and cost-containment

- Cost-containment plans

● Legal Environment:

- Limitations on IPAs/EPOs/PPOs

- Existence of freedom-of-choice and/or mandatory plans

The methodologies employed to collect the types of information delineated above are typically drawn from marketing research techniques. Focus groups, for example, may be valuable in exploring physician attitudes regarding PPOs. If physicians are already sophisticated and involved in PPO development, it can be useful to design and administer a questionnaire which will elicit information concerning current alternative delivery system activities, interest in the proposed PPO, group practice participation and established referral patterns.

Telephone or personal interviews are generally more productive than written questionnaires in obtaining industry and insuror data. Chambers of commerce and the state's insurance department are valuable sources of information regarding the marketplace and may be utilized to supplement the interviews.

Essentially, the market research technique employed will be dictated by the nature and composition of the group to be queried, the availability of information from secondary sources, and the specific type and complexity of information sought.

The development of this market assessment is intended to answer several questions which are essential to the successful development of the PPO. Some of these questions include:

- What geographic area and employers do member hospitals serve and how are they changing?

- What are the present and future employment patterns which would influence PPO usage?

- What are the employer/insurer characteristics that would most influence PPO development?

- What PPO attributes would be most appealing to employers, insurers, and physicians?

- Who are the major brokers and consultants influencing health insurance arrangements and employer benefits design?

• Who else is considering developing a PPO in the specific market area?

• What are the competitors' strengths and weaknesses, and what threats and opportunities do they create?

• What potential market share and profitability does a PPO hold for member hospitals?

In answering these questions, the analyst should extensively use existing data available through professional associations, coalitions or chambers of commerce, local and state governmental or planning agencies, member hospitals and physicians offices, and other secondary sources. This use of secondary data is a very cost-efficient methodology for abstracting information necessary for laying the foundation for a PPO. Once a clear understanding of the local marketplace has been achieved, this information should be presented to the PPO's management decision-making body. This body can then determine the appropriate course of action within the parameters it sees fit for the development of the PPO. With the presentation of the facts for the development of the PPO in the decision-making body's hands, the activities necessary for the market assessment have essentially been completed. The next phase of the feasibility analysis process is that of the organizational assessment.

The organizational assessment should entail a review of the operations internal to the participating hospital and physicians' offices, particularly as they relate to issues relevant to PPO development. The assessment should also include an analysis of the appropriate organizational structure needed to successfully operate a PPO, given a single hospital or multi-hospital system orientation.

One of the essential issues which should be addressed in the organizational assessment is that of physician recruitment. To be successful, the PPO must have a sufficient base of physicians to service prospective payors. As such, it is necessary to determine the attitudes of the medical staffs towards PPOs. It is also important to determine to what extent physicians will discount their services in the PPO setting or establish alternative payment programs that will provide for a more competitive structure within the PPO arena. Discounts or other alternative reimbursement methodologies may be a necessary prerequisite to contracting with an insurance payor. The composition of solo practitioners versus group practice physicians should be identified, as it is more expeditious to recruit group practice clinics into a PPO arrangement than it is solo practitioners. In addition, the nature and extent of existing referral patterns will provide insight as to key physicians to recruit and the feasibility of a closed referral network. As in any other organizational endeavor, it is essential to identify the formal as well as the informal physician leaders, as they will provide a key stimulus to the development of the PPO and can spearhead physician recruitment activities. Through these leaders, it is also possible to establish committees to screen physician applicants and identify the most appropriate participants for the program.

Another significant issue which must be addressed in an organizational assessment is that of utilization review. The utilization review component is indeed the cornerstone of the development of any successful PPO. As such, a thorough evaluation of the review processes in PPO participating facilities should be conducted to determine their feasibility for PPO application. One of the issues to consider in making this assessment is to determine to what extent non-Medicare review is being performed today. The extent to which the review component is addressing privately insured patients at the present time can facilitate the applicability of the review program to the PPO. How extensive is the current review program, and what results have been achieved through this program? Do the hospitals perform ancillary or appropriateness of admission review? What are the physicians' attitudes toward private review, and how committed are physicians to this practice? Can existing utilization review personnel be used in the PPO's activities or must additional staff be considered? These are all questions which must be answered in order to have a thorough understanding of the review mechanism and how it interfaces with the PPO.

Another general issue in the organizational assessment is identification of current systems' capabilities. The current billing and admitting system's ability to accommodate PPO patients is one factor for consideration. What is the relationship between the billing, admitting, and utilization systems and how can these systems be integrated to accommodate a PPO? Also, is there sufficient administrative support to coordinate internal organizational development of a PPO? The most appropriate role for physicians and hospital administration must also be delineated in the development and management of the PPO. These issues can all be identified through a thorough assessment of the systems and managers operating these systems.

Financial issues and capitalization of the PPO must also be reviewed at this stage. The projected cost for the development and management of the PPO should be considered and broken out in terms of developmental, as well as ongoing, funding. The break-even point necessary to show a positive financial position for the PPO should be tabulated and set as an initial objective. In a related vein, methodologies for hospital and physician payment should be considered and evaluated. The financial system's ability to separate payor classifications for PPO patients should also be reviewed. A final issue necessary in determining the financial impact of the PPO is the exploration of long-range revenue sources.

Several legal issues need to be evaluated and their implications fully understood at the point of conducting the organizational feasibility assessment. These include the nature and scope of state and federal laws governing insurance and corporations that would influence PPO development. Currently, some states have special legislation supporting the development of PPOs, whereas other states are void in this area. The appropriate legal structure to provide the necessary governance, control and management of the PPO should be considered and recommended. The most appropriate legal arrangements between and among hospitals, physicians, insurers, employers, and the PPO should be evaluated and considered within the planning framework. Other legal issues which need to be considered are how the legal structure is affected by anti-trust, the potential level of price-fixing exposure and exclusive contracting. Often, the legal structure of the PPO itself can be arranged such that a great deal of flexibility and control can be maintained by the providers in the pricing of their services. Legal counsel of the sponsoring organization should conduct a thorough review of current statutes and legislation regarding and limiting the development of PPOs to determine the legal constraints which may limit or modify the desired PPO structure or functions.

As a result of this internal organizational assessment, the sponsoring organizations obtain a good perspective on how their strengths and weaknesses fit within their target marketplace. Once these two assessments are matched, a better understanding of the appropriate structure, systems, incentives, and financing arrangements can be understood for the PPO, and a definitive decision whether to proceed in PPO development can be rendered.

The decision to move forward in the PPO planning and developing process should be guided by an objective determination that the proposed organization will be able to reasonably meet predetermined feasibility criteria. These criteria include:

● Prevailing health benefit structures are compatible with a dual option plan.

● Alternative delivery systems, and particularly the PPO concept, are accepted by a significant share of the payor market.

● The payor community is of sufficient size to support a PPO.

● Providers participating in the PPO have sufficient capacity and resources to serve the market.

● Sources exist to capitalize the PPO, and potentially to provide for on-going operations.

● Mechanisms exist and are capable of controlling and monitoring utilization and expenses. This includes, for example, data processing, utilization review programs, and financial systems.

● The proposed provider network will have a marketable competitive advantage.

This may be defined in terms of all or a combination of factors such as price, product packaging, geographical network and consumer access, or recognized provider excellence in the marketplace.

● State and national statutory or regulatory impediments are minimal or can be readily accommodated in the PPO's structure.

Assuming the market and organizational assessments meet these general criteria, management should turn its attention to the identification of PPO development opportunities. Initially, these development opportunities should take form through the preparation of mission and role statements for the PPO as it relates to member providers. Various mission and role statements can be prepared and analyzed in a manner that addresses the problems and concerns of the marketplace and that builds upon the market analysis already performed. These statements should highlight the critical internal and external issues regarding the development of the PPO and provide a framework for management to make an intelligent, planned decision for the future of the PPO.

In developing these statements, it is necessary to have explored alternative scenarios for conditions regarding the PPO. Such considerations will provide management with a better understanding of the potential futures, clarify objective, and eliminate last minute surprises. It is often a good practice to conclude this analysis phase with a planning session or retreat involving the key parties necessary to the successful development of the PPO. This allows all involved to consider, evaluate, and select the most appropriate course of action to develop the PPO. Such a retreat also creates an understanding of the importance of each individual's contribution to the development process, and ensures that the implications of any given decision are understood by all involved. The end product of the examination of strategic alternatives should be a creative combination of facts, judgments, intuitions, and strategies regarding PPO development. This consensus-building phase provides an interpretation and analysis of alternative courses of actions, resulting in recommendations for PPO development appropriate to the marketplace and organization, and a budget for PPO development and operation.

Once the specific structure and design have been approved, it is necessary to determine the steps required to implement this structure. Thus final phase of the PPO feasibility analysis is preparation of a specific implementation plan. In essence, a work plan must be established to guide management in developing the PPO. Although the work plan will be as detailed and as specific as the given level of management determines, at a minimum, the following key elements should be included in the implementation plan:

- Organizational structure and process necessary for implementation.

- Strategies and tasks for implementation.

- Personnel and financial resource requirements.

- Legal and regulatory considerations.

- Medical staff considerations.

- Strategies for marketing.

- Timetable for monitoring, reporting, and follow-up activities.

Once the implementation plan is delineated, the evaluation and assessment process is nearly complete. As with the implementation of any new program, it will be essential for senior management to oversee and spearhead the accomplishment of the delineated tasks and timetable.

The planning and feasibility process identifies the desirability and necessity of establishing a PPO within the confines of any specific marketplace. Naturally, the need for any product must exist before the product is developed. The internal and external market assessments seek to identify the PPO's potential in the marketplace. Through the second phase, organizational assessment, capabilities to meet the need are determined. The third step in the process arrays alternatives for the future of the PPO structure and facilitates consensus on, and selection of, the most appropriate alternatives. The final step in the process provides for a specific, systematic plan which allows the program to be implemented in an intelligent, cohesive manner.

CHAPTER THREE
Organization Patterns

The PPO concept is not as young as it looks.

Although PPOs have attracted much attention in the past two or three years, they have actually been operational in one form or another for a much longer period of time. Perhaps the first generic PPO was the "company health plan" in which an employer had entered into agreements with various providers to provide medical services to his employees. The concept was simple: the physician was willing to discount his fees in exchange for greater volume and expanded market share. Subsequently, we have seen the proliferation of Blue Shield plans, which can also be considered a type of PPO. In this arrangement, a subscriber is given the opportunity to receive medical services from one of a number of designated physicians with no provisions for coinsurance. These beginnings have now generated many more comprehensive and frequently complex arrangements between all participants in the health care spectrum: hospitals, physicians, insurers, employers, employees and third party payors.

Yet, for all the attention that has been paid to PPOs, no uniformly accepted or legislated definition exists. And with good reason. Because of the differing objectives of the PPO, and especially the need to be flexible in dealing with many different elements in the health care spectrum, PPOs have developed much like the automobile industry. Each PPO has a different body style, but as all cars can be used for transportation, all PPOs can be used to deliver medical services. What have developed, therefore, are several characteristics which are almost always found in a PPO. These include, but are not limited to:

1. **Limited and selected group of providers.**
   This may be a grouping of hospitals and physicians or of physicians only, but is virtually never a grouping comprised only of hospitals because of the key role that physicians play in the delivery of medical care. The term "limited" is important, because not all providers can participate (nor would all necessarily want to in a "preferred" provider arrangement). The term "selected" is also important; to succeed, the PPO will have to involve

not only efficient and cost-effective providers, but recognized, quality providers to whom insurance beneficiaries will want to go to for medical services. The entire concept rests on limitation of freedom of choice.

2. **Fixed rates for reimbursement.**
Although it is theoretically possible to establish a PPO by having a different fixed rate for each class of providers, this would be the exception rather than the rule. For PPOs operating in a wide geographic region with differing costs and medical practice patterns, regional rates may be established. These may even vary by volume. Or, the PPO may wish to establish uniform rates throughout its entire service area. The actual method by which providers get reimbursed according to a fixed rate differs greatly. For physicians, it may mean reimbursement according to: a) a percentage of usual, customary and reasonable fees; b) a fee schedule which is frequently based on conversion factors applied to arbitrary relative value study values; or c) partial or full capitation.

For hospitals, it may mean reimbursement according to: a) charges or a percentage of charges; b) per diem by type of service or an all inclusive per diem rate; or c) diagnostic related groups (DRG). (The ramifications and implications of these reimbursement methodologies are discussed in chapter 5.)

The key to a fixed fee schedule is that it gives the payor of health care expenses a method by which those expenses may be better and more accurately estimated.

3. **Utilization controls and other cost containment programs.**
These are necessary to fund the expanded benefits given to insurance beneficiaries to utilize a preferred provider and to remain competitive in the marketplace. Different types of utilization review programs that may be adopted and

implemented by the PPO include preadmission certification, continued stay review, ancillary services review,
review of surgical necessity and preadmission authorization. These different approaches are discussed extensively
in chapter 8.

4. **Economic incentives to utilize preferred provider.**
Insurance beneficiaries must be given a financial choice
when selecting a physician or hospital in a preferred provider arrangement. This most frequently takes place in the
form of eliminating coinsurances and deductibles for the
use of a preferred or designated provider, thus creating
coverage much like that of an HMO. It may also entail
other forms such as expanded benefits coverage for the use
of a preferred provider. For an insurance plan that currently offers first dollar coverage to its subscribers (no out-
of-pocket expenses in the form of coinsurances and deductibles) and wants to implement a PPO type plan, it
would be necessary to redesign the benefit structure to accommodate the appropriate incentives. More often than
not, PPOs are seen as supplement to existing indemnity
insurance.

5. **Consumer choice.**
Insurance beneficiaries must be given the opportunity to
select from a list of preferred providers, or any other provider of his or her choice. The PPO is midpoint on the
continuum between the HMO and the fee-for-service system. If there were no consumer choice, the insurance plan
would more closely resemble that of a health maintenance
organization or exclusive provider organization. Both are
discussed later on in this book.

6. **Rapid claims processing.**
One of the benefits a provider derives from participating in
a PPO is the prospect of quick payment for services. This

is particularly true for hospitals, whose average account in accounts receivable may well exceed seventy-five days. It is of significant, albeit lesser, importance to physicians, especially to the extent that a physician accepts assignment of benefits for a significant number of patients. By participating in a PPO, the provider is essentially accepting assignment. There should be appropriate assurances that the provider is reimbursed in a prompt and expeditious manner.

Types

Because of the diversity in the types of arrangements which may exist in a PPO setting, it is not surprising that a number of different types of PPOs have come into being. Essentially three types of PPOs are recognized, each based on the impetus behind their formation.

1. **Provider-based.**
   This may take the form of a grouping of physicians or of physicians and hospitals. A hospital, in conjunction with participating physicians from its medical staff, could form a PPO organization and enter into agreements with self insured employers or insurance companies. The same could be true for a grouping of hospitals, either independent providers or members of a multihospital system. A key point: *the extent of geographical coverage of the provider-based PPO will determine the interest of the employer or insurer.* For example, an insurance company with beneficiaries located across a significant area in a number of large cities may not be interested in contracting on an individual basis with a PPO comprised of one hospital and its medical staff.

2. **Payor-based.**
   This type is sponsored by the payor and insurer of the

health benefits coverage. It may be an insurance company, a self-insured employer or a health benefits trust covered under ERISA. In this arrangement, the payor holds a contract with individual providers and has a very high degree of control over the network.

3. **Entrepreneur-based.** In this arrangement, a third party holds agreements with both the insurance payor and the provider. An organization that provides administrative services for the payment of insurance claims (such as a third party administrator) is most likely to develop this type of PPO. It tends to be the most geographically restricted.

The specific form which reimbursement takes depends on the sponsorship and other operational policies adopted by the PPO for a payor sponsored PPO. After a provider renders medical services to a covered individual, the bill will be sent to the insurance payor directly. The same would be true for an entrepreneur-sponsored PPO. However, a provider-sponsored PPO may elect to collect the claims initially to perform medial necessity review to adjust provider charges to negotiated amounts or to collect data relating to the provision of services by its members. Outpatient utilization information is crucial to the extent that it provides the PPO with a means to evaluate the performance of its providers. It may opt to collect this data before sending it to the contracting payor. Other data needs are discussed more extensively in chapter 8.

Specific organizational structures are presented in Appendix A.

HMO and EPO comparison

Because of the intense interest being generated in PPOs, and because PPOs are in many respects the fee-for-service response to the recent successes of HMOs, it is only natural to examine the similarities and differences between PPOs, HMOs, and the latest entry into the alternative delivery scene, EPOs or exclusive provider organizations.

A *health maintenance organization* (HMO) is an organized health care delivery program that provides medical services to subscribers on a pre-paid basis. In other words, in exchange for an amount of money which has been agreed upon in advance, the HMO agrees to provide all necessary medical services from the prescribed list of benefits to those individuals who choose to enroll. Three types of HMOs exist:

1. a staff model wherein the plan employs the physicians;

2. a group model wherein the HMO contracts with a group of physicians organized for the sole purpose of providing medical services to a defined HMO population (such as the Kaiser Health Plan which contracts with the Permanente Medical Group); and

3. the IPA (independent practice association) model wherein physicians in private practice, either individually or collectively, contract with the HMO for the purpose of delivering health care services to a defined population, while maintaining their fee-for-service practice.

An *exclusive provider organization* (EPO) is a grouping of fee for service providers who have agreed to provide medical services to a defined group of individuals at a negotiated fee. In this arrangement, the beneficiary has no coverage outside of the network of contracting providers. (Provision may be made, however, for emergency services.)

One of the most critical elements to the understanding of the differences between a PPO and other alternative health care delivery systems has to do with the concept of risk. Because a PPO is an alternative to a normal indemnity insurance program, most PPOs in the development or operational stages do not pass on risk to the provider. Physicians are reimbursed on a fee-for-service basis; as a physician provides care to a covered individual, he or she bills the insurance payor and is reimbursed according to the negotiated fee. Hospital reimbursement methodology is beginning to incorporate more creative approaches that involve some degree of risk. Although hospitals may be paid according to actual billed charges or a percentage of billed charges, it is becoming increasingly more common for PPOs to adopt per diem pricing or a diagnostic related group (DRG) basis. Under a per diem basis, rates of reimbursement are based on either a specific amount for each day a covered patient is in the hospital, regardless of the quantity of services utilized, or may also be based on the type of service being provided, (i.e., medical, surgical, ICU, CCU, obstetrics, pediatrics, etc.). Under the second type of arrangement, payment to the hospital would be based on the number of days an individual was in the hospital and the number of days the patient received a particular service. This type of arrangement also involves risk because reimbursement is based on the *negotiated rate,* not on the *quantity* of services provided. Adoption of this methodology will obviously have an impact on the physician recruitment strategy adopted by the PPO.

Health maintenance organizations, on the other hand, are successful *because* they place the provider at risk. For example, in an IPA-type HMO, reimbursement is based on a capitated amount. A capitation pool is normally established, and the pool is credited based on the number of people enrolled. The amount can be based on the number of men, women and children or can be based on contract size (one party, two party, multiple-party). Physicians may then be paid on a modified fee-for-service or a capitation arrangement. The point is that the money in the capitation pool is all of the money available to pay for medical care. Because of the contractual arrangements, if the quantity of care exceeds the available dollars, the level of reimbursement is simply reduced.

An EPO is similar to a PPO when considering the concept of

risk. Providers are generally reimbursed on a fee-for-service basis, and the risk remains with the insurance company, not the provider. Thus, regardless of the quantity of services provided, the providers will be reimbursed according to the negotiated rates. It should be noted that although both the PPO and EPO may accept risk on a limited basis, they have strong incentives to be cost effective. Unless they can demonstrate cost savings, they will not continue to be designated as preferred providers, thus losing the benefits that the arrangement would bring.

Provider selection by the participant and coverage outside of the designated network are two other significant areas to be discussed when comparing these three alternative delivery systems. In a PPO plan, the covered subscriber has a choice between using a designated or "preferred" provider (with expanded benefit coverage) and using any other physician of his or her choice (usually with a coinsurance and deductible). A financial incentive has been created for the member to utilize certain providers, but coverage is maintained, albeit at a lower level, when a nondesignated provider is used. The term "swing" is frequently used to describe a PPO plan because the subscriber has the option of using either a preferred or non-preferred provider on a case-by-case basis throughout the enrollment year.

Just the opposite is true in an HMO or EPO setting. After enrollment into the plan, the subscriber is limited to the physicians he or she may select. Some HMO or EPO plans may require the subscriber to select a specific physician and hospital and utilize them on an exclusive basis, while other plans may be more flexible to the extent that the subscriber is free to go to any contracting provider. One of the main differences comes with the requirement that the subscriber has no coverage outside of the designated provider network for a non-emergency situation. Usually, the subscriber is "locked in" for the enrollment year and may not switch to another insurance program except at open enrollment. This is in stark contrast to the PPO, which provides coverage even when a non-designated provider is used.

Another area of difference has to do with the flow of money. An HMO collects premium dollars and disperses a portion of that income to providers based on a negotiated rate. In this sense, the HMO functions as an insurance company because it performs the underwriting and claims payment functions. However, this is not necessarily the case in a PPO. Because the insurance company already has an established underwriting and claims processing system, the provider-based PPO does not usually incorporate these functions into its operations. If the PPO were to do this, it would be in direct competition with the insurance payor, something which would not enhance the objectives of the provider-based PPO. An entrepreneurial-based PPO is slightly different, especially if formed by a third party administrator. Because third-party administrators (TPAs) are essentially the claims-payment function for one or more insurance payors, the entrepreneur-based PPO may well provide this service to its clients, especially if the insurance companies, self-insured employers or similar companies for whom the TPA already provides service participate in the PPO arrangement.

The provision of marketing services is another area of difference among alternative delivery systems. Marketing is generally tied into the underwriting function. Thus, in an HMO, the plan markets its own services. However, in a PPO or EPO, the underwriting and hence the marketing is usually done by another entity. For example, a provider-based PPO which contracts with an insurance company to provide medical services to the subscribers employed by certain companies will not market its provider network. This function will be carried out by the insurance company. Obviously, one exception to this would be a payor-based PPO.

Finally, legislation is another area that will point up differences among HMOs, EPOs, and PPOs. In 1973, Congress passed Public Law 93-222 which was the enabling legislation for HMOs. Aside from establishing requirements for benefit coverage and other criteria for operation, the law also provides that

HMOs should be able to require an employer of twenty-five or more employees to offer an HMO option to employees if more than twenty-five of the employees reside within the service area of the HMO and if required by the HMO to do so. This gave HMOs tremendous leverage in the marketplace and is frequently cited as a prime factor in the success of many HMOs.

This is not the case with PPOs. No national legislation deals with the subject. Nor, as noted earlier, is there any formal definition. Some states have passed enabling legislation for PPOs and EPOs. For example, in California, the state legislature passed three bills in 1982—the first steps in regulating the PPO and EPO industry within the state. California law requires provider-based PPOs to have authorization from an insurance company or an employer before finalizing the provider network. It also provides for the establishment of some utilization review mechanisms. But these two factors are not nearly as encompassing as the previously mentioned federal legislation, or for that matter legislation enacted by many states to regulate the HMO industry.

Organizational structures and issues

A myriad of types of structures can be adapted by the PPO. Among them:

1. unincorporated association;
2. partnership;
3. for-profit corporation;
4. professional corporation;
5. financial joint venture between providers;
6. tax exempt organization;
7. taxable non-profit corporation; and
8. cooperative.

These models apply primarily to the provider-based PPO mode. The PPO established by the payor or entrepreneur will most probably be developed as a separate but related line of business and therefore would not necessarily require the establishment of a separate entity. It may also choose to form a subsidiary company such as Aetna has done with its "Choice" program. Dependent on such things as risk and financial considerations, the payor or entrepreneur may well want to establish the framework of the PPO outside of the existing organizational structure.

The ultimate organization and governance of the PPO will have a strong influence on how the PPO will be funded. This issue is central to provider-based PPOs, rather than insurance company or entrepreneur-based PPOs.

Selecting the appropriate structure for the PPO will be based on a number of factors. The nature of the provider community may well be the prime determinant to the organizational structure. Such things as the extent to which physicians are organized in group practices or IPAs will have a strong influence on the adopted structure. The capital requirements and potential sources of funding necessary to start the PPO will also have a strong impact on the form the PPO will take. Similarly, the extent to which the PPO will be taking on financial risk will play a significant role.

A number of organizational issues should be addressed by all parties, not only in the development of a PPO, but in the operations as well. Some of these issues include:

- the role of providers in the PPO,

- the method by which providers will be recruited,

- the extent to which the PPO complies with legal requirements, especially in the area of antitrust,

- the tax exemption status of the PPO,

- the structure of the PPO to limit corporate liability,

- the method and level of funding,

- the extent to which the structure will provide for flexibility, particularly in the areas of provider participation and contracting with insurance companies,

- the nature of the contract between the payor and provider, particularly with respect to:

  - claims payment

  - utilization review

  - contract termination

  - resolution of disputes, including grievance and arbitration

  - third party liability

- The extent to which the PPO is at risk for the medical care being delivered by the organization, both financially and legally.

Governance

The specific form that the governance will take is directly related to the type of PPO formed, as well as the parties involved and the control that each brings to the table. For example, an insurance company that has formed a PPO may well do so within its existing corporate structure and merely consider it a different line of business. The same is true for the entrepreneurial model.

Because of the dynamics of the relationship between physicians and hospitals, and between providers and the marketplace, a provider-based PPO must be sensitive to these factors in the development of its governance. In a provider-based PPO, which has as its members both physicians and hospitals, it will be critical for the governance to address the needs of all parties. If it does not, the level of participation may not be appropriately balanced. For example, physicians will probably be very reluctant to participate in a PPO they perceive to be hospital controlled, without a substantial level of physician representation.

The specific form of governance also will be dependent on the organizational form adopted. A joint venture between a hospital and its medical staff may have equal representation of both physicians and hospital administration. A cooperative venture between providers and an insurance company will have different representation in its form of governance.

In any event, the governance of the PPO will have to address several critical issues discussed elsewhere in this book. Some of these issues are:

- What will be the service area of the PPO?

- If the service area covers a wide geographic area, how will the diverse interests of the participants be represented, and at what level will issues be decided?

- Who will decide the eligibility criteria for membership in the PPO and who will apply those criteria?

- What utilization review programs should be adopted?

- How will the criteria for the utilization review programs be developed and applied?

- What will the strategy be for the development of criteria for contracting with insurance payors?

To be successful, the PPO must address these and other issues pertaining to network development and the ongoing management in such a way as to meet the needs of its members as well as those entities with which it seeks to do business.

CHAPTER FOUR

Provider Participation

Despite the recent publicity received by PPOs, the fact remains that providers—both hospital administration and physicians—do not have a full and complete understanding about the mechanics of a PPO.

Because a PPO is an alternative delivery system, it is not uncommon for providers to confuse this concept with that of an HMO. This seems particularly strange when considering that PPOs in many respects are a response by fee-for-service providers to the successes of HMOs. Before a PPO can operate effectively, the participants must be educated relative to the concepts involved and completely aware of the policies and procedures of the PPO.

Certain environmental factors must also be in place before a PPO can operate. The prime factor here is competition. In geographic areas with an oversupply of physicians and hospital beds, it is very likely that at least one PPO is in the developmental stages, or perhaps even further along. However, it is possible that in certain areas competition is not perceived by the providers. As noted earlier, there are very few, if any, compelling arguments for providers to join a PPO where there is no perceived competition. Also, in communities with no competition, it is virtually impossible for a PPO to operate. For example, in a town with only one hospital and a grouping of physicians with relatively full practices, there will be no incentives for the providers to change the status quo. The areas most susceptible to the development of a PPO are the sunbelt states, yet PPOs are developing in other competitive areas such as Denver, CO, Minneapolis, MN, and other selected areas in the Northwest and Mid-Atlantic states.

A provider-based PPO which is essentially hospital controlled will have to give great thought to the nature of each hospital's relationship to its medical staff during the education and recruitment processes. Historically, there has been an adversarial relationship between hospital administration and the physicians on staff at the hospital. *If administration is unable to win support for this concept, the PPO has virtually no chance for success.*

It is important to assess how hospitals and physicians *individually* perceive competition. For example, a hospital may think that it functions in a very competitive environment and want to develop a PPO as a competitive strategy. However, the medical staff of that hospital may not have the same perception and thus may not be motivated to become involved in an alternative delivery system such as PPO.

The approaches that an administrator might take to communicate the concept to the medical staff can vary from individual meetings with key, influential members of the medical staff to a general meeting with all members of the staff. Ultimately, the approach adopted will be dependent on the nature of the relationship of the administrator to the staff, the confidence of the physicians in hospital administration, and the various environmental factors discussed above.

The formation and implementation of a PPO can be a powerful tool for an administrator, especially if the PPO is hospital based. In this type of plan, the administrator is generally responsible for recruitment. As such, he can use participation in a PPO as a carrot to attract new physicians, or as a reward to loyal physicians already on staff.

The extent to which hospitals and physicians participate in the development and operation of the PPO is also dependent on its sponsorship. A PPO sponsored by an insurance company is likely to have little provider input into policy areas. But a provider-sponsored PPO will likely have complete control by physicians and hospitals, with little initial input by the insurance payor.

Selection criteria

An element very critical to the long-term success of the PPO deals with the criteria established for provider participation. To ensure the viability of the PPO, it is necessary to select providers who are efficient, cost effective and maintain high-quality standards. This is especially true for the provider-based PPO, which will most probably be asked by an insurance company what standards it can identify that guarantee the quality of the network.

Abstract concepts such as quality are always hard to quantify. Yet, it is a process which every provider-based PPO will have to go through if it expects to be in business for any period of time. Some of the criteria for physicians' participation that may be established include:

1. current state license;

2. professional liability (malpractice) insurance in specified amounts;

3. staff privileges (which may be defined as active rather than associate, provisional, or courtesy) at a preferred hospital;

4. the absence of any action by any state medical quality assurance agency in which the physician has practiced or is licensed to practice medicine.

One of the reasons to stipulate professional liability insurance is to protect the PPO financially in the event of legal action taken against a PPO physician.

The criterion of staff privileges pertains not so much to quality as it does to ensure that the participating physician can and will admit patients to a PPO hospital. A physician who cannot meet this criterion does not serve the member hospitals, nor can patients going to this physician receive the full inpatient benefits of the PPO plan as there will most probably be a co-insurance and deductible for the utilization of non-designated facilities.

It is incumbent on the PPO to develop and maintain physician provider profiles so that it may establish subsequent criteria for physician performance.

It is much easier to develop objective criteria for hospital participation which can be used to ensure the quality of the network. Some of these criteria include:

1. state license;

2. professional liability insurance;

3. accreditation by the Joint Commission on Accreditation of Hospitals;

4. specific service capabilities which may include the following services:

    —Anesthesia
    —Clinical Laboratory
    —Dietetic
    —Medical
    —Nursing
    —Pharmaceutical
    —Radiological
    —Surgical
    —Coronary Care
    —Emergency Medical, Standby
    —Intensive Care
    —Intermediate Care
    —Nuclear Medicine
    —Occupational Therapy
    —Outpatient
    —Physical Therapy
    —Rehabilitation Center
    —Respiratory Care
    —Social Service
    —Speech Pathology and/or
    —Audiology

5. financial viability, which may include such things as debt service, percentage of occupancy, and Medicare and Medicaid volume (and any other information which is available through public documents);

6. status as a general, full-service, acute-care institution;

7. cost (theoretically, it is possible to operate a successful PPO with cost-effective institutions and physicians without

discounts, the acceptance of risk, or even utilization review (UR) programs, *if* the cost of care through those providers is less than a PPO with significant controls).

The PPO may also use its UR programs to support the argument of a high-quality network. By establishing rigid criteria for each of its UR programs, as well as to having specific programs established for quality assurance, the PPO can objectively defend the quality of its network. A key component of any UR program is the definition of medical necessity and how this definition is applied and implemented.

Developing selection criteria

A significant and sensitive issue must be faced by the PPO in terms of application of the selection criteria with respect to the recruitment process. The PPO has a choice in applying any criteria on a prospective or retrospective basis. For example, a hospital administrator who is recruiting members of the medical staff to participate in a PPO may develop and apply criteria before approaching physicians. The advantage to this approach is that problems in weeding out inappropriate providers are eliminated. However, this same administrator risks alienation from the medical staff as all are not invited to participate. Although it may be more politically advantageous to apply the criteria retrospectively, it can also lead to potential utilization problems. This is a real catch-22 type problem, with no known solution. An insurer-based or entrepreneurial-based PPO may already have historical utilization data against which it can evaluate potential providers.

Regardless of the time frame within which the criteria are developed and applied, it will be imperative that the criteria be uniformly applied to all prospective participants. The adopted criteria, therefore, cannot vary from doctor to doctor or hospital to hospital. Although PPOs as yet have not been subjected to rigorous legal scrutiny, a PPO that does not uniformly apply membership criteria would be subject to potential legal attack based on state or federal antitrust grounds. A more complete discussion of legal issues may be found in chapter 9.

Conditions of participation

To ensure a viable organization, the PPO will want to establish some conditions or requirements that providers would be expected to meet. Regardless of the type of PPO involved, there will be some contractual document between the provider and the payor. This document will identify performance standards by both parties. For some PPOs, there may be Articles of Incorporation and Bylaws to which members are expected to conform.

The PPO may wish to adopt Rules and Regulations or similar standards. Also, it may want to require financial participation in the form of an application, initiation, or membership fee. These need to be clearly delineated in the document(s) which bind the provider to the PPO.

Recruitment strategies

In planning recruitment strategies, it is necessary to examine the environmental factors and determine the extent to which they may be sufficient to support the development of a PPO. Also, it is imperative to know that the program parameters are going to be sufficient, not only at a level to attract providers, but also at a level to attract the providers who are wanted. For example, a PPO may establish a specific level of reimbursement for its providers which is low for a given geographical area. This PPO may well have no problem in contracting with providers, but more likely than not they will be physicians who are new in the area or just out of medical school and not the medical staff leaders whose support is most helpful in both the development/ planning and operational stages. Obviously, if the environment will not support the operation of a PPO, it makes little sense to initiate one.

Payor-based and entrepreneur-based PPOs find it most easy in dealing with established provider networks in setting up a PPO plan. This is true for a few key reasons. The first has to do with ease in recruitment. The entire process can be expedited because one agreement provides access to a provider grouping. The agreement may be with a provider-based PPO, a multi-hospital system, an independent practice association (IPA) or grouping of IPAs, a medical group or a separate corporation which has been established by a hospital and its medical staff as a joint venture. The possibilities are limitless.

Another consideration is the historical lack of knowledge and adversarial relationship between the insurance payor and the medical provider. Because the insurance industry has little knowledge regarding what makes a physician or hospital administrator tick, it is much easier to leave this task for someone else. It is important that there be an understanding up front as to the expectations and quality standards/criteria to be used. It would be infinitely more cumbersome for the payor or entrepreneur to become knowledgeable about the provider community and then to go about entering into agreements with providers on an individual basis. However, some PPOs like Admar's Med Network in Southern California, prefer to have individual relationships with providers in order to maintain control.

There is a much different set of circumstances in dealing with the establishment of a provider based PPO. If it is to be a PPO whose membership is composed exclusively of physicians, it is necessary to have support and leadership from another physician or group of physicians who are respected in the community. Physicians respect and listen to other physicians. On the other hand, if the PPO is to include both physicians and hospitals, it is crucial to have the active and vociferous support of hospital administration (as well as physicians). Physicians need to know that their hospital is involved and supportive of the concept. It is impossible to recruit otherwise. In terms of recruiting other hospitals, it is most helpful to have another administrator involved in the process. Somewhat like the physicians, hospital administrators are most apt to listen to other administrators.

In recruiting physicians, essentially three different approaches can be employed. The first is to work with medical groups, either general practice, multispeciality or speciality groups. This provides access to a maximum number of physicians with a minimal amount of contact. This must be supplemented with other recruitment activities, because a successful network must have multiple delivery sites in order to attract patients. Although it may be necessary ultimately to have physicians sign individual applications or agreements, the ease and expediency in dealing with a medical group administrator may prove substantial. A second approach is to recruit the open staff of a hospital. This would most probably be done through a general meeting. Unless handled properly and with great care, and unless the administrator has been active in previously educating the medical staff, there is a potential for disruption by a few physicians. Finally, the administrator may wish to work with physicians on a selected basis. This may take the form of individual or small group meetings. An insurance or entrepreneur-based PPO seeking to develop its own provider network (as opposed to contracting with a provider-based PPO) may wish to adopt the above strategies. As noted elsewhere, the insurance company or entrepreneur may well have utilization experience which may be used as a tool in this process.

Here are some key points to bear in mind during the recruitment process:

- The recruitment process needs to be sensitive to the normal referral patterns of a defined medical community. If a primary care physician cannot refer a patient to a specialist with whom he or she is accustomed to working with, the potential for the physician to participate is diminished.

- There should be general parameters about the mix of physicians wanted by specialty, including total numbers. Obviously, as the potential user population gets larger and more geographically dispersed, so should the provider network.

● Demonstrated support by participating providers is critical during the recruitment process. Physicians listen and react to other physicians, and similarly with hospital administrators. The development of a hospital physician network may well hinge on the support given by hospital administration, and on the administrator's ability to effectively communicate the program concept.

● Strategies for physician contact include general medical staff meetings, group physician meetings, individual meetings, and meetings with medical groups.

Networking

As noted earlier, a multi-site PPO is going to be much more appealing in the marketplace than a single site PPO. To that end, a provider-based PPO may wish to link up with other PPOs in order to be more attractive to the purchaser. This is an example of the case where bigger is potentially better. Also, the same principle applies to a multi-site PPO that wishes to have greater geographical coverage.

A PPO wishing to network should consider the following points in advance:

● Will joining another PPO enhance their own position in the marketplace? If so, to what extent?

● Is the nature of the network consistent with the goals and objectives of the PPO?

● Is the new entity going to be financially viable? To what extent will financial support be necessary?

● Is participation in the new entity going to be financially justifiable?

- Who will have control of the organization? If there is to be a board of directors, how will it be elected?

- How will the individual components of the network participate in the negotiation of an agreement with a payor?

Service mix

In developing a PPO, it will be necessary to provide or arrange for the provision of comprehensive inpatient and outpatient services. If the services cannot be provided within the PPO setting, the patient will then be forced to seek care outside of the system and all benefits will be lost.

At the same time, however, it should be clearly understood by all parties that a PPO will not be able to provide all medical services. For example, one hospital may not have any neurosurgeons on its staff and, therefore, cannot provide this medical service. However, this is where the appeal of the PPO comes into play, because the patient may still receive covered medical care by going outside the network. As noted before, the higher the frequency of this type of action, the lower the success of the PPO.

The types of physicians that a PPO will want to recruit will depend in part on some of the policies that govern the operation of the PPO. For example, a PPO program that adopts the "gate-keeper" system requiring a covered patient to go to a primary care physician first (usually defined as family practice, general practice, obstetrics/gynecology, pediatrics and internal medicine) will want to weigh its recruitment in this area more so than a PPO that does not have this requirement.

Here are the physician specialties usually found in a PPO plan:

- Allergy

- Anesthesiology

- Cardiology

- Dermatology
- Endocrinology
- Family Practice
- Gastroenterology
- General Surgery
- Internal Medicine
- Neurology
- Obstetrics/Gynecology
- Opthalmology
- Orthopedic Medicine
- Otolaryngology
- Pediatrics
- Pulmonary Medicine
- Urology

As noted earlier, the hospital should be able to provide a wide range of medical services; these were listed earlier in this chapter under the heading selection criteria.

Impact on providers

Unfortunately, virtually no empirical evidence will give a provider, hospital or physician, any indication of what the impact of joining a PPO will be. If a PPO type plan was offered to an employee group, it is possible (though not probable) that all or none of the employees would choose to select a preferred provider. It is also thought that a percentage of those employees electing to utilize a preferred provider will be selecting their regular physician, and won't create any new business. It is important during the recruitment process that the PPO not be presented as a panacea, for there is no way to accurately predict what the level of utilization will be.

Regardless of their base, PPOs must develop the management information and data systems necessary to produce information relating to the utilization of services. In time, PPOs should also be able to project the percentage of penetration or utilization they can expect to achieve.

CHAPTER FIVE
Finance

The successful financial management of PPOs requires effective planning and organization in the areas of capitalization, operating revenue, and provider payment methodologies.

The incorporation of capital needs into the PPO's business and financial plans is best accomplished through *pro forma* capital expenditure statements. Exhibit 5.1 identifies and organizes the typical capital expenditures necessary for a provider-based PPO.

Any new business enterprise requires some level of initial capital to fund the enterprise's long-term financial needs and the working capital needs until reasonable levels of operating revenues are achieved. The PPO as an enterprise requires little initial capital relative to other businesses.

The services and purpose of the PPO should identify the parameters of financial requirements. For example, PPOs whose primary purpose is to organize providers and negotiate rates require little capital. In contrast, however, PPOs that provide extensive claims processing, claims auditing, utilization review, and plan management services usually require sophisticated data processing abilities and will demand a much larger level of initial investment. This example identifies a key component of a PPO. *The purpose and services of the PPO must be clearly defined prior to any investment.*

The organization sponsoring PPO development must thoroughly understand the market to be served and define a purpose that fits this market's needs. This definition of purpose or mission should serve as the beginning of an overall business and financial plan. These plans are the mechanism for identifying capital need and may serve as a prospectus for investors.

Typical initial capital requirements for provider-based PPOs include the cost of initial organizational meetings, one-time communication materials, legal fees, and utilization review system develoment. Other capital requirements more typical in nonprovider based PPOs include claims system development and benefit plan design. Although specific amounts can only be determined on a detailed case-by-case basis, the authors' experience suggests that provider-based PPOs require from $300,000 to $500,000 in initial capital.

Exhibit 5.1
Pro Forma Capital Requirements

Organizational Development
    Legal Fees $
    Travel Expenses $
    Meeting Expenses $
    Printing $ _____

    $

Systems Development
    Utilization Review System $
    Quality Review System $
    Membership Tracking System $
    Claims System (Optional) $ _____

    $

Market Development
    Initial Advertising $
    Brochures $ _____

    $

Working Capital (For Development Phase)
    Accounts Payable $
    Salaries $ _____

    $ _____

    _____

TOTAL CAPITAL NEEDS $ _____

Selecting the capital source

The sources of PPO investment capital are typically providers, payors, or independent entrepreneurs-investors. In addition to the relative advantages and disadvantages of each capital source, a primary consideration must be the motives for investing in a PPO. These motives often determine how rapidly growth will occur and to what extent costs are controlled. Providers often invest as a defensive strategy to preserve their current patient base. A hospital considering a PPO arrangement may well ask its medical staff to participate financially, depending on the attitude of the medical staff and the physicians' perceptions of the environment as competitive. Payors, on the other hand, see the PPO as a mechanism for controlling their costs. The opportunity to make money is a typical motive for independent investing and is the case with entrepreneurial sources of PPO capital.

Although the sponsoring organization by its mere existence may dictate the source of capital, the extent to which the capital source can be selected may greatly influence the PPO's long run viability. This selection becomes more important as one considers the often conflicting objectives in the PPO, i.e., containing costs while increasig utilization. Since final control resides with the PPO's owners (those providing capital), the source of ownership ultimately determines the objectives to be achieved. The particular characteristics of the market served and how well the ownership's philosophy and objectives match that market will predict the likely accomplishments of the PPO.

The legal structure of the PPO should also be considered during the process of identifying the capital requirements and sources. Although the legal structure does not affect the amount of capital needed, it can greatly influence the ability to attract investors. The ownership status (for-profit versus not-for-profit), the investor's level of financial risk and control, and the investor's level of participation in profits will determine the type of party investing capital in the PPO. As such the most appropriate investment opportunity should be structured to attract the type of investor that would cause the PPO to be successful.

Generating operating revenues

A second financial area is that of generating operating revenues. The ongoing support of a PPO can come from many different sources. A key principle in determining the most appropriate source of operating revenue is to again look to the PPO purpose.

The purpose of a PPO can be viewed from the perspective of who benefits from the arrangement and who gains the value added to the marketplace as a result of the PPO. From this perspective, those who benefit and gain significant value should fund the PPO's operation.

Exhibit 5.2 illustrates the function and benefits resulting from the PPO in the marketplace. This is one method for beginning an analysis of the most appropriate sources of PPO operating revenue.

Many provider-based PPOs function as a "broker" for member providers. To the extent that a brokerage function is performed, the broker is always paid by those they represent, and as such, this type of arrangement is most appropriately funded by member providers. The level to which the PPO adds value to the marketplace, however, should be funded by the payors who purchase services through the PPO.

Either approach to ongoing funding is appropriate, given the PPO's purpose. But one methodology must be selected. If the PPO's purpose indicates that provider funding is most appropriate, one methodology to generate the revenue is to charge member providers for the cost or the cost-plus-a-profit for the PPO. A second methodology is to withhold a percentage of the claim paid to member providers as a source of revenue to fund PPO operations.

In those cases where payor funding is more appropriate, a typical approach is to charge the payor a flat rate per covered life per month. Another method used is to charge a percentage of the total health insurance premium for PPO services. Few PPOs are charging on a per claim or per occurrence basis, although that is a viable option.

Exhibit 5.2
Paradigm of PPO Marketplace Functions and Benefits

PPO FUNCTIONS	BENEFITS	
	PROVIDERS	PAYORS
A. Provider Brokerage	● Increased Marketshare	● Convenience
	● Convenience	● Expediency
	● Increased Profits	
B. Negotiate Rates	● Negotiating Strength	● Expediency
C. Select and Organize Providers	● Can serve multi-site payors	● Expeciency
		● Convenience
		● Identifies efficient providers
D. Perform Utilization Review	● Policing Peers	● Control utilization
		● Control costs
E. Process Insurance Claims	● Track performance	● Monitor/evaluate costs and utilization performance
		● Convenience

Regardless of the method used to procure operating revenue or its source, it is essential to budget the expenditures and revenues necessary to operate the PPO. Although this level is relatively minimal in many cases, it is prudent financial management to control the PPO's financial operation.

The sample budget identified in exhibit 5.3 provides a framework for organizing the financial operations of the PPO. This is an example of a provider-based PPO with a relatively narrow range of services and functions.

Payment methods

The last major financial issue in PPO management is the method and process for paying member providers. Current practice has most providers using current payment methodologies and simply discounting the rates charged. This approach, however, does nothing to alter the practice of health care treatment in a manner which makes the system more efficient or effective.

Any methodology used to pay PPO providers should ideally instill financial incentives to be efficient and effective in the provision of medical care. This method would also reward those providers who are efficient and not reward the inefficient.

The consideration of the best method for paying providers should also include the compatibility of the payment method with the claims processing systems used by payor clients. The ultimate test of the payment method selected is its ability to be administered. A second consideration is to achieve significant predictability and stability in the cost generated by the PPO. To achieve this result, member provider's rates should be fixed for a time period—probably one year.

Three alternatives for paying hospitals will be considered and their advantages and disadvantages are outlined in exhibit 5.4. One alternative is to use the traditional process of hospital billing and simply discount the total hospital charge per bill. This

Exhibit 5.3
Sample PPO Budget

Revenue
    Membership Fees $ _____

          Total Revenue $ _____

Expenses

    General and Administrative
        Office Rental $
        Telephone $
        Printing $ _____

    Salaries
        Administration $
        Provider Relations $
        Marketing $
        Utilization Review $ _____

    Travel
        Provider Relations $
        Marketing $
        Utilization Review $ _____

    Data Processing $ _____

    Advertising $ _____

          Total Expenses $ _____

Exhibit 5.4
Hospital Payment Methodologies

Method	Advantages	Disadvantages
1. Discounted Charges	• Initial payor price break	• No performance incentives
	• Discount level easily determined	
2. Per Diem Rates — Comprehensive — By Service	• Offers performance incentives	• Hospital assumes risk
	• More predictability in pricing	
3. DRG	• Costs more accurately reflect resource utilization	• Hospital systems not yet operational
	• Offer performance incentives	• Claims systems not yet compatible

discounting approach may offer some initial price break to the payor, but it does not offer any incentives for the hospital to be more efficient. Furthermore, discounted charges do not provide any assurance that the price charged will be any lower than it would be outside the PPO.

A second method for paying hospitals, which is being used by the State of California in its Medi-Cal contracting program, is the use of per diem rates. Per diem rates can be comprehensive and all inclusive, thus covering all services offered by a single rate. Per diem rates can also be established by medical service offered. The use of by-service rates minimizes the level of financial risk the hospital assumes; however, under either approach the hospital assumes the risk of managing their costs within the per diem charge. As such, the per diem approach, either all inclusive or by service, instills incentives for efficiency.

A third method for paying hospitals is to negotiate payment on a DRG basis, utilizing the hospital's information systems as necessary to comply with future government reimbursement practices. Although this method may prvide better management information and the opportunity to control costs more efficiently, commercial health care payors do not yet have the claims systems to pay providers under this approach. As PPOs further develop, it is likely that the DRG payment methodology will be more often employed.

Physician payment in the PPO can be provided through several different mechanisms. These mechanisms are identified below and displayed in exhibit 5.5.

Physicians who participate in PPOs are often paid through a discounted charge process similar to that used in hospitals. This process often uses a negotiated percentage of the payors claims profile for usual, customary, and reasonable rates. The typical level of payment has been observed to be between 70 per cent and 90 per cent of Usual Customary Rates (UCR) in many areas.

A second physician payment process is to use a fixed fee schedule that identifies a fixed amount to be paid for each medi-

Exhibit 5.5
Physician Payment Methods

Method	Advantages	Disadvantages
1. Discounted Charges	● Easily administered	● No performance incentives
		● No consistency in individual rates
2. Fixed Fee Schedule	● Provides consistency and predictability in rates	● May not reflect variation in cost
	● Easily administered and compatible with claims system	
3. Full or Partial Capitation	● Offers performance incentive	● More difficult to administer
		● Not readily accepted by physicians

cal procedure performed. Many states use a Relative Value Schedule (RVS) for paying workers' compensation claims.

This RVS identifies a unit value for each medical procedure, with the unit value multiplied by a conversion factor to determine the total price per procedure. The negotiation and setting of the conversion factor can easily create a fixed fee schedule that is widely understood by member physicians. For most major payors, processing claims on a fixed fee schedule basis poses no particular problems.

A third approach is to pay physicians on a full or partial capitation basis. Although the authors are not aware of any particular PPO which pays physicians on this basis, the capitation offers an additional incentive to be cost efficient by placing the physician at risk for the care provided.

A concluding issue related to provider payment concerns the link between provider payment and utilization review decisions. Although utilization review is discussed separately, it is mentioned here since it is critical to link these two functions in order to provide a strong control over the appropriateness of care provided by the PPO. To date, the most effective method for changing provider habits to be more efficient appears to be to place the provider at financial risk or to link provider payment with review decisions.

CHAPTER SIX
Marketing to Payors

True PPO marketing, like the marketing of any other goods or service, mandates that all planning and decision-making center on the problems, concerns, attitudes, and behavior of the consumer, who must be satisfied with the particular product.

All useful academic as well as practical definitions of marketing focus on the consumer (client, buyer, customer—the one who "receives" the goods or service). For PPO marketing, there are several consumers: hospitals and physicians are consumers of the PPO from the provider's perspective; insurers, employers, and trust funds are the primary PPO consumers from the payors' perspective. The beneficiary or subscriber of a health plan which contracts with a PPO is also an additional consumer. For purposes of this chapter, we will focus on marketing the PPO to the payors of health care services. To the extent that the other previously mentioned consumers impact payor marketing, and they assuredly do, they will be presented.

The payors of health care services (insurance companies, self-insured employers, ERISA trusts and third-party administrators) have become a common, general definition of the PPO consumer. PPO management's ability to solve effectively this consumer's health care problems will be one measure of PPO success. PPOs that indeed solve consumer's problems add value to the marketplace, and so long as they maintain this added value, PPOs will continue to be a viable component in the health care delivery system. Once the marketplace no longer recognizes a value from the PPO, PPOs will no longer exist as they did before. They will either alter their purposes or fade into oblivion.

Market analysis

Successful PPO development and marketing must begin with a thorough analysis and understanding of the consumer the PPO intends to serve—the health care payor. Furthermore, this analysis must be specific to the geographic area served by the PPO, although general payor trends and patterns can be helpful.

A first step in analyzing the payor market is to determine the size, shape, characteristics, and behavior of payors. Payors' health care problems that can be addressed by the PPO must also be identified. *Throughout the process of assembling data on the payor, the analyst should continually attempt to identify those payor characteristics that separate payors into distinct unique groups.* This separation can then be used later in the process to develop the PPO's marketing segmentation strategy.

Common payor demographic characteristics that should be researched are identified in the list below. These characteristics tend to describe the size and structure of a given payor market. The variables are also interrelated. In collecting data to complete these type of profiles, secondary data sources such as the Chamber of Commerce, the State Insurance Commissioner, the Department of labor, and various other public and private sources can be most helpful.

Payor Demographic Profiles

Insurers

- number of health insured lives
- location of insured lives
- per cent of business that is indemnity; per cent that is ASO
- average account size
- size of sales force and type of sales force
- market share by health premium dollar
- typical benefit plans offered
- average account duration
- brokerage and consulting firms commonly used

Employers

- number of employers by workforce size
- number of dependents
- concentrations of employee residences
- number of self-insured/self-administered employers
- number of self-insured/ASO or TPA-administered employers
- number of indemnity insured employers by carrier

- typical levels of deductible and co-insurance
- benefits of consulting and brokerage firms used

Brokerage Firms

- types of clients
- major insurers represented
- lines of business
- influence over benefit plan design
- role in claims processing

Trust funds

- number of members covered
- concentration of members' residences
- claims processing arrangement
- level of benefits coverage
- number of dependents

An additional critical aspect of the market analysis is the identification of the payors' problems with that of the health care delivery systems. The escalation of health care cost has been the major issue of concern for the past several years. As cited in the Jan. 10, 1893, issue of *Business Insurance,* insurers are predicting average rate increases in group health insurance for 1983 to be 25 per cent to 35 per cent. This will be the third consecutive year for such increases. With cost increases a major concern, the ability of the PPO to provide long-term as well as short-term approaches to controlling costs makes it an attractive vehicle to be integrated into payors' health benefit plans.

Costs, however, are not the only problem confronted by payors. Access, mix of services and programs, appropriateness of services delivered, and quality of care provided are also major issues. Few, if any, major payors are willing to sacrifice the quality and integrity of medical care for cost purposes alone. Most major payors have simply indicated that they expect reasonable, quality care at reasonable prices. *The elimination of unnecessary and inappropriate care is a major focus to resolv-*

ing the problems payors have with the health care delivery system.

An issue related to the identification of payors' problems is an assessment of how, if at all, these problems are being resolved today. To an extent, approaches available in the marketplace that are alternatives to PPOs in the resolution of payor problems, are competitors to the PPO.

At the current time in the evolution of PPOs, HMOs appear to be the only practical competitor. Other PPOs, as they develop, become competitors as well. A profile of the competitors, their strengths, weaknesses, range of services, pricing arrangements, cost control mechanisms, and other salient aspects that are of value to the payor should be considered and evaluated in the assessment of the PPO marketplace. As the competition for a specific PPO becomes more refined and sophisticated, a more thorough analysis for the competition and marketing approaches to combat or divert competition must be developed. Although there are currently few places in the United States where competition between PPOs actually exists, it is likely that competitive postures will be taken in the near future as this delivery form further develops.

Payor related profile

The previously collected demographic data assists the marketing analyst in understanding the fundamental structure and nature of the local PPO marketplace. This analysis is necessary, but it is not sufficient for a comprehensive market assessment. Another specific payor related profile must be developed. This profile should focus in on the attitudes, opinions, plans, and desires of health care payors in a given marketplace. Such a profile provides variables that are not easily obtained from secondary data sources but are critical to establishing a sound market assessment.

Payor attitudinal information is best collected through interviews with a sample of health care payors. Methodologies used in collecting this type of information can be either personal interviews, telephone interviews or focus group interviews. All of these methodologies can be effective depending on the specificity of information desired. Regardless of the methodology selected, it is important to collect such information based on payor size and type. By collecting and categorizing these attitudinal variables by payor size and type, the analyst can more effectively group payors and their attitudes into separate, unique market segments.

A final component in the market data collection is an identification of the influential decision-makers in the purchase process for PPO services. Since in many respects the employer is the ultimate buyer of health care services, it may be wise to begin the assessment of decision-makers with the employer. An initial review of all employers will indicate that influential decision-makers exist internal to the employer organization as well as external to the employer.

As with any organization, a natural political and bureaucratic hierarchy exists within the employer's management structure. In marketing the PPO, it is critical to understand this hierarchy of decision-makers that participate in the health care purchase.

For major Fortune 500 corporations, one will typically find a personnel manager, benefits manager, employee relations manager, medical director and possibly several other individuals, usually within a human resources division, who will have some active role in this purchase decision. In addition, a phenomenon of recent years is for the company president and occasionally the chairman of the board to become involved in establishing corporate strategy and direction for health care cost containment. This phenomenon has occurred simply because health care costs have grown to represent such large portions of corporate expenditures. For sound corporations, this phenomenon has been extended to include the hiring of health care managers whose job it is to purchase services.

In assessing decision-makers external to the employer, it is essential to understand the nature of the insurance marketing process and what parties become involved in influencing and delivering health insurance products. Parties involved in this process typically include the insurer, broker, brokerage firm, consulting firm, third party administrator and potentially the health care cost containment consultant. Of this list of characters, the insurer, brokerage firm, and benefits consulting firm tend to be the most influential parties. The market assessment must analyze which brokerage firms tend to represent which insurance carriers and how the brokerage firms market the carrier's product to the employer. Often, the benefits consultant will be involved in recommending a given insurance carrier's product as well. Although the third party administrator and cost containment consultant may take a role in influencing the decision-making process, they typically are not as influential as the other parties.

The critical aspect of this part of the process is to identify how the various external parties influence each other and influence the employer's decision. Collecting this type of information may be difficult, as it often hits to the heart of these players' marketing strategies. However, through interviews with various brokerage firms and various employers, the marketing analyst can develop a keen sensitivity for who is most influential and how this influence is exerted.

Once all of the demographic, attitudinal, and behavioral data has been collected, the analyst must break down this data by characteristics that tend to group the payors into separate, unique market segments. The ability to break out payors into unique segments will ultimately enhance the total marketing process for the PPO. Ideally, the marketing analyst should develop market segment profiles that indicate how these variable group payors relate and how these segments can be affected by the PPO's marketing program.

Product development

Following the assessment of the marketplace, a second phase to the marketing process begins—the actual product development phases. From the assessment of the marketplace, the marketing analyst can provide a reasonably clear indication of major payors' problems and how the PPO arrangement may be able to address and resolve these problems. The organization of the PPO's salient components around marketplace problems is probably the most significant development aspect of the entire process. Given this concept, the PPO membership and organizational structure should be configured in such a way to best meet payors' needs. As with the development of any product, it is often difficult for management to look outside of its own internal needs to that of the marketplace; however, the ability to make this external assessment materialize into a bona fide product is extremely critical at this point.

Once the concept and structure of the PPO have been fairly well defined, it is wise to take the concept to various payors and request their opinions of the structure. Modifications can then be made to the initial concept and structure, given the opinions and assessment of the payors reviewing the approach.

In reviewing the PPO concept with payors, be sure to clarify who would be the most logical party to fulfill many of the insurance-type functions. These functions include the processing of claims, underwriting the insurance risk, designing of benefit plans, and marketing to individual subscribers within groups. Although in some marketplaces it may be appropriate for the PPO to perform some of these functions itself, it is wise to assess the marketplace and determine who is the most capable and qualified for each of the respective functions, rather than attempting to build unfamiliar expertise within the PPO itself. Furthermore, the PPO should maintain the flexibility to contract with several different types of entities which could and will perform these insurance functions.

Throughout the product development process, it is necessary to build confidence not only with the marketplace but with the providers represented as well. A typical phenomenon is for payors to want and expect provider groups to be completely organized and formed prior to being approached. On the other hand, providers often expect the PPO to have contracts arranged with payors before they will be willing to commit to the PPO. This particular phenomenon tends to be the rule rather than the exception in PPO development. It often becomes necessary to develop letters of intent or commitment on behalf of both buyers and sellers to establish the PPO arrangement. PPO managers must develop initial step-by-step confidence building with both their provider members as well as payors. The process for this confidence building can be the letter of intent approach previously identified. Other mechanisms, however, should be investigated as well and used where appropriate to develop the confidence of both payors and providers.

Component testing

The components of the PPO must also be clearly defined and developed. These components most notably are the specific providers, their range of services and locations, the cost control mechanisms employed in the program, the extent to which the PPO becomes involved in the handling of any claims, and any other specific component that is appropriate for a given marketplace. These components, although addressed in other portions of the book, should be clearly defined and tested prior to initiating the program in any aggressive sales manner. To test these components, provider-based PPOs have the ability to use their own organizations' employee health plans as a testing ground for the PPO itself. Where this is not feasible, selecting employers who are willing to experiment may provide the opportunity to test all of the PPO systems prior to offering the program to the general marketplace. This step of program testing is vitally

important, since most marketplaces do not easily forget or for-
give mistakes made by an organization.

Market segmentation

At this point in the process, we have assessed and evaluated
our market and designed and developed our PPO. Now comes
the time for developing strategy on how we get the PPO to the
buyer. One of the first steps is to break down the total payor
market into unique, separate market segments. The process of
segmenting the market allows the marketing manager to organize the marketplace into separate distinct groups that have common characteristics and behavior. Once the market has been organized in such a fashion, it is much more effective to identify
a specific segment or segments that the PPO wishes to approach
rather than to attempt to satisfy the entire market.

Insurance risk

Later on we will discuss the various characteristics that can be
used to segment the PPO market. However, at this point, it
would be wise to look at who truly assumes the insurance risk
for a defined market. The organization that is liable for the insurance risk of a given patient population is usually the most
important organization in the PPO purchase process. As such,
this is often a reasonable criterion for segmenting the market. By
separating the market into those separate, unique organizations
who assume the insurance liability, more distinct segments can
be identified.

Using the element of insurance risk assumption as our char-
acteristic for segmenting a given market, many segments are
easily identified. Insurance carriers are a common market segment. Within the carrier segment, it is important to identify carriers who provide primarily indemnity health insurance versus
those that are primarily administrative services organizations.

For the carrier offering a large base of indemnity health insurance, the PPO will desire to contract with the carrier directly. For carriers that offer primarily administrative services, the PPO will wish to use these carriers as a mechanism for contracting with the carriers' clients.

Another segment is that of the self-insured employer. Self-insured employers must organize some methodology for processing claims. Those that administer claims themselves are typically more fully informed and more in control of their health purchase decision than any other particular market segment. Thus self-insured, self-administered employers are often the ideal segment if they are large enough to support a broad-based PPO. Employers who use the services of third party administrators or have an administrative-services-only arrangement with an insurance carrier are typically slightly more removed from the purchase decision and will have slightly different attitudes from the self-administered employer.

Although the insurance carrier and self-insured employer are often the ideal market segments for a PPO, one should not overlook the union trust funds, multiple employer trusts (MET), or governmental bodies. Each of these particular segments has its own unique advantages and disadvantages in a given marketplace. Regardless of the segment(s) selected, a local market decision is necessary; no broad generic approach will fit all communities. Other characteristics that can be used to segment a given market include client size; whether the client is local, regional or national in scope; the extent of benefit coverage; the union status of employers; and many other aspects that can help break down a large market into smaller components.

To evaluate the feasibility of the market segments identified, consider the following two questions:

- Is the segment capable of being reached?

- Is the segment large enough to be profitable?

For those market segments that answer both of these questions in a positive manner, one must prioritize the segments according to profitability and develop strategies for approaching each particular segment.

Market approaches

In approaching each particular market segment, it is important to understand the role of the various parties in the health care selling/buying process. In many respects, the PPO salesperson must be very well versed in health care, health care cost-containment approaches, the insurance industry, benefits design, and the administration of health insurance plans. The primary role of the PPO salesperson will be to represent the PPO to many diverse groups interested in acquiring the PPO's services.

Throughout the selling process, the PPO salesperson undoubtedly will be in contact with many independent insurance brokers and major brokerage firms. The broker and brokerage firm play a vital role in the distribution of insurance and insurance products since they typically search for the most economical insurance product for a given employer, and they often take an active role in recommending approaches to insuring given risks. In some of the larger brokerage firms, claims administration and claims processing are functions that they perform themselves. Often, the ability of the PPO to affiliate, or possibly to undertake a joint venture with a brokerage firm, can greatly expedite the marketing and sales of the PPO.

Two other organizations that can typically take a role in the distribution of the PPO are benefits consulting firms and third party administrators. Through the benefit consultant's role in organizing and designing health benefit plans, the PPO will become a likely alternative which can be structured into the array of approaches available. Third-party administrators (TPAs), on the other hand, typically have a full book of clients for whom they are processing claims. Whenever the TPA can identify approaches, which will save clients money, it assuredly will. Furthermore, large reputable TPAs can be an excellent party with whom the PPO could joint venture to provide a comprehensive delivery system coupled with claims processing and administration.

Other organizations that will not take an active role in purchasing PPO services but that should be kept informed of PPO development include: insurance trade associations, benefits management groups, and local business coalitions. Although these groups will not make decisions regarding the purchase of PPO services, they are an excellent forum for presenting the PPO alternative and they are a good conduit for keeping key purchasers informed of your development.

Presenting the program

By now we have evaluated our market, developed our PPO, identified our target market, and determined how we can best approach that market. Our next step is actually presenting the program to a given payor and negotiating the PPO contract. Before any specific contacts are made, it will be necessary to establish all the necessary brochures, sample contracts, presentation material and any other promotional tools used to sell the program.

Once promotional materials are assembled, one can begin to approach the specifically identified target clients. Try to obtain an introduction or lead from a familiar party to a prospective client. If this is not possible, one must simply contact the client and request a reasonable amount of time to present the program. It is critical to communicate clearly how the program works, what it is, and possibly more important, what it is not. After there is a clear understanding from the buyer as to what exactly you are offering and how specifically you wish it to work, it will become necessary to discuss the components of a specific contract that would be held between the payor and the PPO.

In negotiating the PPO contracts with payors, maintain a great deal of flexibility in terms of how the PPO will function. The essential component is to organize a contract that will allow the providers to benefit from increased patient volume and the payors to benefit from some approach to containing costs and providing quality care.

Since the PPO is new in many areas, it is difficult to push for closure on a contract at an early stage. It is better to gain a little bit of commitment than none at all. As time progresses with a potential client, it is much more reasonable to push for closure on a given contract.

Summarizing the marketing plan

Although this chapter has outlined many components essential in marketing the PPO to payors, the total framework for analyzing and structuring these issues should be the PPO marketing plan. The main components of a PPO plan already have been discussed in one form or another throughout the chapter. However, at this point, the structure for a marketing plan will be outlined to assist marketing management in organizing their thoughts. The PPO marketing plan should consist of the following components:

- Situational analysis
- Marketing objectives
- Marketing strategy
    - product design
    - pricing policy
    - promotional program
    - sales approach

- Tactical plan

- Market monitoring/evaluation

The situational analysis for the marketing plan is essentially the market assessment with which we started this chapter. After your situational analysis is completed, it is necessary to establish marketing objective for the PPO. These objectives can be the number of contracts consummated for a given year, the number of enrollees to whom the PPO is available, or possible claims paid or premium dollars flowing through the PPO. *What is essential is that the objective be time-limited, specific in responsibility, and measurable.* Throughout the time period, management can continually monitor the ability of the program and its marketing arm to achieve these objectives.

It obviously is important to have a clear marketing strategy. One essential component is the product design itself. As formerly discussed in the market assessment and product development sections of this chapter, we have structured a methodology for designing the product to best fit a given community. Once this product has been structured, its design becomes a critical component to the marketing strategy. To the extent that there is flexibility in this product design, the PPO marketing arm can alter the product slightly to better meet the needs of specific clients.

A second component in the marketing strategy is the pricing policy. Since the pricing of the PPO is discussed in the financial chapter, we will not elaborate on it now. However, it is necessary to note that the sensitivity of given payors will differ by segment, and this should be incorporated into your strategy. Pricing policy should reflect the value that the given payor receives from the PPO itself, not necessarily the cost incurred.

The final components of program promotion and sales tend to be closely linked. The *promotion program* should clearly identify and emphasize those components that are critical to the given payor market segments. The *sales approaches* for the PPO are fundamentally those approaches that best use the current marketing channels that are effective in the distribuution of the insurance product.

The tactical plan essentially defines who does what and how in order to implement the strategy to achieve our objectives. The tactical plan should be specific to the objectives and strategy outlined. *For all practical purposes, the tactical plan is essentially the management by objectives to implement the marketing program.*

As with all other management functions, marketing management must continually monitor and evaluate its performance and ability to achieve the objectives outlined in the plan. As such, mechanisms should be established in the planning phase to monitor the processes and achievements. Once these systems have been established, the PPO marketing manager can monitor the performance and continually evaluate the approaches that will make the PPO a successful product in the marketplace.

CHAPTER SEVEN

Cost Management/Utilization Review

In the short term, PPOs probably can get started based upon the acceptance by a contracted purchaser of the theoretical advantages of negotiated prices and a competitive approach to the market. But, over time, it is clear a PPO must prove itself to be truly price competitive if it is to survive and prosper.

At this stage, few, if any, PPOs can demonstrate actual savings to either consumers or sponsoring payors. And both need to be convinced that they are getting their money's worth.

From the consumer's viewpoint the nature of price competition in health care should increasingly parallel that in other industries. Higher price levels where they occur can be tolerated where there is also a desirable non-economic quality in the goods offered. Health care product differentiation is to some degree already perceived by consumers today, as seen in such areas as over-the-counter drugs where price leadership can reflect consumer acceptance of brand names and associated quality.

In areas where multiple choices are offered, consumers, in considering alternate insurance plans, differentiate not only between such characteristics as price and share of costs, but also on such product elements as ease of access and community status. Preference for a particular practitioner and desire to utilize a specific site of care is also an element of product differentiation affecting choice of coverage. The convenience and amenities aspects of health care programs, however, can be expected to have less importance as financial incentives begin increasingly to favor cost as the major element in a subscriber's selection of a health insurance plan. For emerging PPOs, however, the more critical sale is to the sponsoring organization and/or insurer.

It is important for the new PPO to demonstrate that it has organized its delivery system around providers that have a history of fiscal prudence and conservatism in the use of service. These characteristics are essentially comparative by their very nature and difficult to establish except in the broadest sense from generally available data. In some instances, to be sure, a major payor may have accumulated and can access comparative data in reviewing a particular provider's cost and use patterns. In others, government data acquired through a claims payment system or a required reporting program may also be available.

Prudent provider network design suggests inclusion of lower cost alternative delivery vehicles such as surgi-centers, ambulatory care programs, and home health agencies. These delivery vehicles, however, may not be included in the payor/sponsor's benefit package and will need insurer sponsorship for inclusion in specific contracts.

Another element of network design that can be cost controlling is minimizing PPO development and operational expenses. Organizing the network around existing processes and proven, cost effective systems in processing of claims, accumulation of data, reporting of information, and overseeing of utilization may be highly cost effective and, it should be noted, can build ties to strong organizations that can lend market credibility and support to the new PPO.

Evaluating cost controls

Once network design and system choices have been made with an eye to minimizing potential costs, the PPO must establish vehicles to control the costs generated in the actual provision of service. In measuring the effectiveness of the PPO's cost controls, it is possible to use as a yardstick the experience of HMOs and insurance/indemnity plans in the PPO's area(s) of operations.

Regardless of the payment system, ultimately the nature of the individual provider's cost patterns will control the PPO's ability to compete and thrive under the rigorous demands of a price sensitive market.

An institution will need to assess its ability to render each of its programmed services on a cost effective basis within its service specific zone. This does not mean that only the low cost, high volume services will be affected but that each service will have to be cost competitive in its unique demand market in order to prosper. Over time, experience should be comparable to that which has occurred in deregulated industries where cost competition can be initially hazardous but ultimately advantageous to the efficient survivor(s). *The ideal outcome should be one in which sufficient numbers of competitive structures insure efficiency in utilization without producing price insensitive monopolies in a given market area.*

A PPO's competition can be expected to derive from other financing and organizational schemes, including traditional fee-for-service systems, with minimal formal linkages between payor, provider and patient; HMOs with maximum linkage; and PPOs with their more moderate open arrangements.

The traditional fee-for-service system will find it most difficult to develop price competition if such vehicles for cost controls are not organized and easily recognized in the market. Revenue limitations based upon declines in business volume are a likely outcome for the isolated providers and would occur because of a competitive loss of market share and failure to develop an effective business strategy. PPOs offer such providers a defensive strategy against such business loss.

Internal cost controls will require that hospitals develop ways to relate costs to specific services and to gather competitive price data in their markets. Having achieved cost efficiency, the institution needs a collective vehicle—such as a PPO—to put forward its products and services in most market areas.

A PPO's financial arrangement with a contract payor should expedite payment and build up operating cash reserves. These reserves can produce a decline in the cost of money, and have potential for generating non-operational interest income.

Even in a situation that supports strong internal controls and administrative efficiency, the PPO, once it is price competitive, must also be able to demonstrate an ability to control utilization of services. A key criticism of some PPO models is that they may cancel the effect of lower costs and prices with off-setting incentives designed to increase utilization beyond that which is truly appropriate and necessary.

One of the many problems that a PPO must face has to do

with the fact that no inherent incentives control cost. Although revised program design is addressing this issue, early design with respect to reimbursement was based on a discounting methodology that served only to encourage inflated costs. Only recently have PPOs begun to adopt the concept of the acceptance of risk by participating physicians. Heretofore, risk was a concept associated exclusively with health maintenance organizations, thought to be the antithesis of the fee-for-service system. In fact, one of the recruitment techniques and selling points of a PPO is that it offers the fee-for-service physician a competitive model to the HMO.

It is imperative that PPOs develop comprehensive cost management programs for a variety of reasons. Without such programs, increase in utilization (both on an inpatient and outpatient basis) will offset price discounts traditionally offered by PPOs. Also, insurance payors will be faced with the same problems that they face today: rapidly inflating health care costs and little if any ability to predict the costs. Simply put, if the PPO cannot contain costs, it will not be meeting its primary objective and, thus, will not be in business for long.

Cost containment must include other approaches than just discounting, for discounting does not address the fundamental issue of utilization. As Arnold Hussman, benefits manager for Atlantic Richfield Company and Chairman of the Employer's Health Care Coalition of Los Angeles, points out, "I am not so interested in discounts as I am in efficiency. I'll make out better in the long run if I can avoid the doctors who hospitalize my employees at the drop of a hat."

It is important in this discussion to differentiate between the terms *cost containment* and *cost management*. In many respects, cost containment is a misnomer because it is simply not possible to contain costs in the truest sense. One need only to look at cost escalation caused by improved technology and inflationary increases to understand that cost containment, *per se,* is virtually impossible to achieve. It is possible, however, to "manage" costs. This is carried out by developing the appropriate parameters for the delivery system itself, as well as incorporating appropriate reimbursement incentives. Cost management may also be achieved by ensuring that appropriate and necessary services are consistent with the level of care to be delivered. The goals and objectives of the PPO should be established with the above distinction in mind.

To develop an effective and credible cost management program, it is first necessary to do two things. One has to do with an assessment of how the system currently works. Each area of the country will have different systems, conversions and policies for provider reimbursement. It is necessary to have a clear understanding of these interrelationships in order to take a second step, which is making appropriate changes.

Two key cost management components

Cost management activities traditionally fall into two categories: reimbursement strategies (physician fees and hospital charges) and utilization review (outpatient and inpatient). In the world of a fee-for-service Medicare, reimbursement is usually based on charges or a percentage of charges. In this system, the provider it not at risk for the cost of care being provided to the patient. There are not built-in incentives for efficiencies or economies of scale, in fact just the opposite. Providers tend to spend more (through providing more extensive procedures, ordering more tests, confining patients longer in the hospital, etc.) because they are rewarded for both high charges. In other words, the physician and hospital are typically paid more if they charge more.

Several new reimbursement methodologies are currently being considered or implemented as part of a cost management strategy in the fee-for-service system, encompassing also preferred provider organizations. These methodologies, discussed in detail in other chapters, include per diem, capitation, and DRG-based charges. The advantages offered are simple: it places the provider at risk, and it forces the hospital to pay closer attention to the delivery of ancillary services. The disadvantages are not quite so obvious. Adoption of these reimbursement programs will mean that the hospital may have to contend with medical staff politics, as well as some provider dissatisfaction at the prospect of being placed at risk.

Financial incentive programs are another area that can substantially impact a cost management program. First, implemented in a pre-paid or HMO environment, financial incentive programs seek to influence the medical practice patterns of physicians by providing monetary rewards for the delivery of cost efficient medical care. Usually, these programs are based upon the premise that many inpatient procedures and tests are amenable to outpatient settings, representing a significant level of savings.

One of the methods of implementing a financial incentive program would be through a redesign of provider payment methodology or a redesign of employee benefits. For example, an insurance company could pay physicians at a higher level for selected procedures if performed on an outpatient basis. (A listing of such procedures may be available through the county medical society, a local foundation for medical care or a regional Blue Cross Office.) In fact, one PPO in California is being developed along this premise, except that it is requiring its physician members to perform a list of procedures on an outpatient basis, unless otherwise medically indicated. Another approach might be to lower or eliminate the coinsurance for outpatient utilization of services. Unlike the first approach, this focuses on the employee rather than the provider. These approaches make it worthwhile for all participants. The insurance payor should also come out ahead because more expensive hospital inpatient admissions did not occur.

A second financial incentive program that the PPO may wish to adopt is the creation of some sort of a retention pool. Under this arrangement, a sum of money, taken out of premiums or provider payment, is set aside in a trust account. Goals for provider performance are negotiated and agreed upon in advance, and funds would be distributed based upon the provider's ability to meet those goals. If goals are met, the pool serves as a reward for cost efficient behavior. If not, it then serves as a type of discount and is returned to the payor. This approach requires a high level of sophistication.

A method must be agreed upon in advance by the providers to distribute the money in the pool. A catch-22 type question then unfolds: "Should a greater percentage of the pool go to those physicians who provided the most services?" In essence, the issue is one of rewarding physicians for efficient performance, and has been one with which many an IPA (individual practice association) has wrestled. Another pitfall in this approach is the prospect of adverse selection or, put simply, the prospect for enrolling an abnormally unhealthy employer group, which may utilize services more than originally anticipated. Should the PPO adopt this approach, it must have the management information systems in place to collect data on individual provider performance on both an outpatient and an inpatient basis. Also, the retention pool must be of substantial proportions so that it can truly provide an incentive for the providers to practice in a cost-efficient manner.

A number of variations and other creative methodologies also may be adopted, depending on the flexibility of the PPO and the insurance payor and acceptance on the part of providers of these approaches.

Utilization review programs

The implementation of utilization review (UR) programs is a second key element to a successful cost management program.

Very simply, UR can be defined as an evaluation system that seeks to determine the necessity, appropriateness, and efficiency of the use of medical services, procedures, and facilities. In a hospital, this includes review of the appropriateness of admissions, services ordered and provided, length of stay (LOS), and discharge practices both on a concurrent and retrospective basis. The inclusion of a UR program into a PPO framework is important for several reasons, not the least of which is the growing sophistication of the health care purchaser.

An effective utilization review system relies on a number of personnel, operating as a team, to carry out all the functions of the system in an efficient and cost-effective manner. They include the attending physician, the review coordinator, the physician reviewer, the discharge planner and the utilization review committee and the quality assurance committee.

The most important health care deliverer remains the attending physician. In spite of the inroads by third-party payors, allied health care professionals and administrative individuals, it remains the attending physician who has knowledge of the individual patient's particular needs and problems. This knowledge is of paramount importance in the process of determining the necessity and appropriateness of medical care. The attending physician is the chief decision-maker regarding what is really needed by the patient. And, therefore, the physician's interaction and meshing with the review process is of critical importance.

To review the cost and quality of patient care delivered, the methods by which utilization review is accomplished are:

(1) **Pre-Admission Review** of elective procedures, which is a medical care review performed to assess the medical necessity prior to the patient's admission to the hospital. Prior authorization (or approval in advance) assures the appropriateness of that admission and further assures that only the patients requiring an acute level of care are admit-

ted to the hospital. Generally, elective surgery and major diagnostic and therapeutic procedures should be performed when pre-operative indications are present. The physician requesting the hospitalization documents the medical indication for the procedure; the medical director reviews the submitted information and assigns a length of stay. The advantage of pre-admission authorization is assurance to all parties of the medical necessity of the procedures and services rendered and cost coverage.

(2) **Concurrent Utilization Review** is an on-going review of the medical necessity and appropriateness of admission and continuous stay in the acute short-term hospital, focusing primarily on the issues of appropriate hospital utilization. It consists of both admission review and continuous stay review.

(A) *Admission Review*. Admission review involves reviewing the patient's medical record, a process to determine the appropriateness of the admission to a level of care in an acute care hospital. Using specific level of care (LOC) criteria—namely severity of illness/intensity of services—the medical record is reviewed within twenty-four (24) hours of the first working day following the patient's admission to the hospital. At the time of this initial review, the review coordinator reviews both the patient's condition and treatment needs at the time of actual review. This type of review is commonplace in the HMO industry. However, physicians in private practice are very sensitive about pre-admission review, and for that reason, the PPO may wish to implement this type of review where medical care has consistently shown to be unacceptable either in utilization or quality.

(B) *Continuous Stay Review*. Continuous stay review involves reviewing the patient's medical record during hospitalization to assess the medical necessity and appropriateness of the continuous confinement at the acute-care hospital level of care. It also includes a continuous assessment of the quality of care being provided to validate that care is being provided at the appropriate level.

The objectives of continuous stay review are:

1. to assure that payment shall be made for hospital level of care (unless otherwise justified);

2. to assure that optimum standards of quality are met; and

3. to assure effective utilization of health care services.

For those admissions or continuous stays which are ultimately deemed to be unnecessary, patients would be advised in writing that they would be financially responsible for care received beyond a specific time and date. One can easily see the necessity of linking the payment process to the utilization review function. If this is not done, the insurance payor will be paying for services which are not medically necessary or appropriate, and the thrust of the UR program as a cost management vehicle will be lost. Admission certification and continuous stay review can be implemented on a concurrent basis for all admissions, emergency and elective.

(C) *Ancillary Services Review* is a retrospective review of those charges which appear on the bill, exclusive of normal room and board charges (namely laboratory and X-ray services). This type of review is in the embryonic states and requires an established and uniform standard of care for which a data base which delineates ancillary utilization by diagnosis, procedure and provider is necessary. Studies have attempted to identify the norm for utilization of arterial blood gases, electrocardiograms and blood chemistries with selected diagnoses during a hospital confinement. After analysis of data, however, meaningful frequency-distribution curves did not emerge. While it is possible to define modal behavior, review of the exceptions beyond the mode has usually shown extenuating circumstances.

Ancillary services utilization has not been effective in identifying targets for physicians. However, over a period of time, the review should be able to uncover ancillary services which were ordered unnecessarily by the physician, charges for ancillary services which were either never reported or never ordered, and, if a per diem reimbursement is in effect, services that should be covered under the per diem rate.

Under the DRG system, prospective payment review of ancillary services usage reports provides a means of quick identification of variant patient care. The key identifier is a high cost center for an individual case or the presence of a cost center not usually utilized within the DRG. This type of variant should be subject to automatic critical evaluation of the patient record.

As stated, this is a retrospective review process of cases or data related to the issue at hand. The data base or study population is derived from cases previously discharged or historical data from previous occurrences.

(D) *Surgical Review.* Surgical review is a retrospective review of the patient's medical records and tissue analysis to determine the appropriateness of surgery. Persistent questions concerning the cost and medical appropriateness of surgery have given rise to several approaches to study and control of the levels of surgical utilization. Unnecessary surgery, also called "surplus," "excess," "inappropriate" or "unwarranted" surgery consists of procedures that are judged to have been performed without sufficient clinical justifications. There are various indicators that unnecessary surgery might exist. However, without accepted criteria to define the need for surgery, validity of the extent of unnecessary surgery cannot be measured and evaluated. Differences in clinical approaches and professional judgments complicates the formulation of such criteria.

These differences are often considered acceptable among professionals and can result in quite variable standards concerning indications for specific surgical procedures. The difficulty of documenting specific instances of unnecessary surgery causes doubts about its existence—hence, the frequent qualification of unnecessary with quotation marks. An alternative to retrospective review of surgical procedures might include such measures as prospective programs of pre-surgical consultations. These programs, commonly called surgical second opinion plans, usually rely on a panel of surgical specialists who evaluate the desirability of a specific surgical procedure when a patient has been informed by a surgeon that an operation is advisable.

Similar to ancillary services review, this is done retrospectively. The PPO should gather data and use it as a method for evaluating performance, if surgical review is included in the UR program.

(E) *Quality Assurance (QA) Program.* The quality assurance program is a means to assess the quality of care in an area of medical practice where actual performance is measured against objective criteria which defines acceptable and adequate practice. A quality assurance program begins with problem identification and ends with sustained problem resolution. Within the scope of this cycle, all recommendations, follow-up activities and monitoring action must be included.

Because this program can be carried out on a concurrent basis with the hospital review coordinator reviewing the chart against established criteria, it means that immediate intervention is possible if deemed necessary. This has a positive effect on the quality of care being rendered to PPO patients.

Because of the prevailing emphasis on cost containment, utilization review may be an area of primary focus for many quality assurance programs. Many routine quality assurance studies that highlight the over utilization or under utilization of resources relate directly to utilization review functions. Moreover, standard monitoring processes and focused reviews may be developed to address utilization review functions, including justification of admission, justification of length of stay and appropriate monitoring of both. Further utilization review activities should cover how the program relates to discharge planning and to actions concerning resource management, both human and monetary.

One of the issues facing a PPO seeking to develop a UR program is that of the personnel to carry out the specific programs. There are essentially three different approaches the PPO may wish to adopt: delegated, non-delegated and partially delegated. In the delegated approach, all UR activities are carried out by PPO providers—physicians and ancillary hospital personnel. One of the advantages to this is the cost compared to the other approaches to review. However, the PPO is subject to criticism because "the fox is guarding the chicken coop." In the non-delegated approach, the PPO contracts with an independent external review organization—a Professional Services Review Organization (PSRO) or similar entity to perform all utilization review functions. Although this alleviates the fox and the chicken coop syndrome, it is much more expensive to operate and may cause some provider dissatisfaction because of lack of involvement and control. Finally, the PPO may adopt a half-way approach or partial delegation that involves a combination of PPO physicians and physicians from an independent organization performing the review. Ultimately, the decision as to the format of the UR program will rest on a number of factors such as provider attitudes and the demands of the payor community.

With the proliferation of PPOs today, it is imperative that PPOs adopt an appropriate program in order to remain competitive in today's environment.

CHAPTER EIGHT
Operational Issues

In many aspects, the PPO can be seen as a triangular relationship between three distinct parties: the insurer, the provider and the subscriber or patient. Each has different needs and priorities, with each party having a specific relationship to the other two parties. The PPO cannot function unless all three parties enjoy a harmonious relationship. If the originally perceived benefits are not being derived at least at the level at which they were promised, the triangular relationship will suffer.

A number of critical organizational and operational issues require careful attention in the formation and day-to-day operation of a preferred provider organization. Many of these issues will, of necessity, predate the establishment of the PPO as an organized entity. In examining operational issues, one need only to look to the benefits to the various participants in order to understand ongoing concerns.

One of the first appropriate steps to determine what some of the potential issues may be is to perform an environmental assessment. Regardless of the sponsorship of the PPO, it will be important to evaluate the internal and external forces which impact on the participants. From an internal perspective, this entails attitude evaluation, an evaluation of sources of support, an examination of market penetration and the functional mix of business as well as other users critical to internal operations. From an external perspective, this necessitates analysis of competitors' market share and current market strategies, and other forces (such as legal issues) within the environment not under direct control.

From the insurer's perspective, the major operational issues—aside from quality and marketability—relate to the cost of the provider network. In other words, is the network indeed generating sufficient savings to offset the expanded benefits given to the subscriber as an incentive to use the preferred provider? One of the shortcomings of PPOs to date is that in general there has been no empirical evidence presented that points to specific cost savings. Everyone from insurance company actuaries to hospital administrators have conjectured that PPOs by virtue of utilization review programs will save money. But the question remains, "How much?"

Insurers have other concerns about the operation of the PPO aside from the potential cost savings, concerns which closely parallel those of the employer and employee. The main area has to do with access and the operation of the network. The following questions need to be answered satisfactorily: Are there sufficient physicians and hospitals to serve the subscribers? Are they in a close geographic proximity? Do the subscribers have any problems in terms of access? Are the appointment and waiting times appropriate? Do the subscribers have any specific complaints? Are the subscribers being treated as regular fee-for-service patients? Should they be? If the response to any of these questions is negative, it will be imperative for the parties to work together to correct the situation.

Providers have a significantly different perspective in evaluating operational issues. The incentives for providers center around patient volume and financial issues. The participating physician and hospital administrator will ask the following questions: By participating in the PPO have I enhanced my market share, or simply converted existing business to a different financial relationship? Are the contracting insurers making payment within the contractual period? Are the administrative procedures established to deal with PPO patients appropriate and not cumbersome? Is the PPO getting utilization data so that it may monitor its providers? Has there been an increase in patient volume, or a better patient mix, to justify the additional expenses incurred as a result of participating in a PPO? If the volume is not at an appropriate level, are there appropriate incentives in the benefit structure to encourage the utilization of preferred providers?

A provider sponsored PPO may have another operational issue to face—ongoing funding. From the payor or entrepreneur perspective, it will be funded through the premium dollars collected. For the provider sponsored PPO, it will be necessary to generate some level of income to support the maintenance of the network. This funding may come from the insurance company through either a percent of premiums collected, a per capita fee, or some other prearranged financial method; it may continue to come from its membership either through a fixed monthly fee for physicians and/or hospitals, or a variable fee used on actual expenses; or it may take form as a combination of both. A provider sponsored PPO, which is funded through assessments to its member providers, is in a unique position because it is in fact the product (medical services) which is being purchased. However, the purchaser (insurance company, self insured employer, Taft-Hartley or multiple employer trust) is not spending any money to buy the product. If the provider network is indeed successful in containing and otherwise reducing the expense of health care, it seems only reasonable that the providers should somehow be compensated and that the network should be purchased by the user.

From the provider's perspective, other operational issues aside from those pertaining to the benefits being derived must be addressed to ensure the long-term success of the PPO. After the environmental assessment, one of the first issues to be examined will be that of medical staff participation. Who are the physicians who will be sought after to participate? Who are the physicians that want to participate? Are there differences between these two groups? This issue will require significant attention by the administrator. Recruitment approaches are discussed in chapter 4.

Significant importance lies in the level of education of each of the parts of the triangle. Many provider-based PPOs experienced start-up problems because of the lack of sophistication of the payor community. With the high level of press coverage accorded to PPOs during the last two years, this lack of sophistication is being rapidly eradicated and is not a continuing problem.

Provider education is not seen as a major problem. However, it will continue to be an issue that needs to be addressed, even in the most competitive of areas. Physicians may not understand the concept, may not understand the reimbursement methodologies and may experience confusion about the differences between the PPO and the HMO. If it is necessary to educate physicians, it will be necessary to use a physician (perhaps the chief of staff of a hospital) or a hospital administrator as "teacher." Physicians will generally always accept, (and for some reason seem to better understand) other physicians. This same role may be filled by the administrator, depending on the relationship with the medical staff.

Two other issues are crucial to the success of the PPO:

1) How will the physicians be organized?

2) How will the physicians be represented?

A lesson learned long ago is that physicians must be made to feel a "part" of any alternative health care delivery system in which they participate, even to the extent of ownership. At minimum, physicians require a voice in operations. Without this participation, the triangle will break and the PPO will cease to function.

The approach taken to "market" the PPO to providers or to recruit providers is an important element. Too often, providers are promised a certain level of patient flow that fails to materialize. The best approach to provider recruitment is honesty. Physicians and hospitals must not be led to believe that the PPO is a panacea that will solve utilization problems. Moreover, physicians must be willing to make decisions that keep patients out of the hospital. Administrators must have the capabilities to identify and recruit those physicians in order to have the core of a successful network. Without this core, there is little hope for a cost-effective delivery system. Although PPOs are, in many ways, a shot in the arm, there is no satisfactory method to determine the number of individuals who *will* use preferred providers within a defined population.

Another issue relative to providers is that of exclusivity. A provider-based PPO, where hospital physician members do not belong to any other PPO, is certainly in an enviable market position. However, this mythical PPO will most probably not be able to contract with a significant number of payors to warrant such exclusivity. Similarly, an insurance company will probably not control enough health-care premium dollars in a specific geographic area to place an exclusivity requirement on providers. In short, exclusivity is an issue which may be discussed, but will not be feasible unless there is control over a significant number of health care beneficiaries.

Another area where a substantial number of issues will arise is the legal area. One of the problems facing the PPO will center around a hold harmless clause in its agreement with member providers. In some states, professional liability insurance carriers will not cover physicians in the event of a malpractice suit for those amounts that a physician has need to hold the PPO harmless. In this case, if a physician was sued and found negligent, the liability insurance carrier would cover monetary damages for the physician, but not the amount necessary to hold the PPO harmless. In this situation, the physician would be financially liable. Thus, if hold harmless language is included in the provider agreement, it will almost certainly raise questions and problems. The PPO may want to investigate the possibility of purchasing its own insurance policy to cover this situation, or simply to delete the language from its agreements. The PPO may also wish to require, as a condition of membership, that member physicians maintain professional liability insurance policies.

The financial area is one critical to the operation and success of a PPO and one which is sure to raise any number of issues. The first and most important is how the issue of development and planning of the PPO will be financed. For the payor sponsored or entrepreneur sponsored PPO, the answer will almost always be that it will be funded out of existing revenues. However, for the provider-sponsored PPO, it poses an interesting issue: Because the PPO will most probably be comprised ultimately of physicians and hospitals, will it be funded by both? To the extent possible, this is seen as the preferred alternative. For physicians, having a financial stake in a venture such as this will make them much more interested in its success. The less desirable alternative is funding solely through hospitals. Depending on the level of developmental expenses and the number of providers involved, this method may be feasible. Should this method be adopted, it will be imperative for the administrator to have substantial interaction with physicians on an ongoing basis to ensure participation.

Another financial area of concern has to do with physicians' perception regarding the level of discounts. In a typical PPO arrangement, physicians may be asked to discount their charges up to 20 per cent and perhaps more, depending on their level of charges relative to their peers. However, hospital discounts are usually significantly less, even if converted to a per diem or DRG form of reimbursement. The basis of cost computing is completely different for a hospital. It will be important for this to be clearly communicated to physicians to avoid any negative feelings or attitudes toward the PPO. A complete discussion of financial issues may be found in chapter 5.

Finally, regarding financial issues, the reimbursement methodology must be given serious attention. Specific approaches are discussed elsewhere in this book. Reimbursement methodology will impact the recruitment process.

Information needs

As any PPO becomes operational and begins providing medical services to specified groups, it is imperative for the appropriate information systems to be established and for providers to understand the provisions of each agreement the PPO has entered. The need is obvious: if a provider is unaware of how to function in this new environment, there is virtually no chance for the success of the PPO.

Every provider in the health care spectrum participating in a PPO arrangement has informational needs, some more so than others. There is a critical need to ensure proper patient identification. It is important for several reasons:

1. To ensure, as a patient is admitted to the hospital, that the

patient account is properly established. This is especially true if the hospital is at partial risk through a per diem or DRG-based reimbursement system. This is also important with respect to the financial reports to be generated by the hospital and the PPO to monitor financial performance.

2. To ensure that the patient is subjected to the provisions and terms of any utilization review program.

3. To ensure that, in the event of an emergency, the appropriate physician is called.

Patient identification can take several forms. Ultimately, it will be dependent on such factors as the size of the group to be covered and the relative sophistication of the insurance company in this area. Some of the options include a plastic ID card, a special sticker for an existing insurance certificate or some other form of specially printed ID card. This may be supplemented with an eligibility roster or a special phone number that the provider may call to certify eligibility and benefits. One of the problems inherent in this system, as with others, is the means by which the plan ensures the person authorized to use the insurance benefits is actually the one using them.

Providers have other significant informational needs. Every individual coming into contact with a patient, or in any way involved in the administrative aspects of the delivery of medical care to an individual covered by a PPO-type plan, will need to be made aware of the terms of coverage. Experience has shown that provider unawareness creates confusion and dissatisfaction in any alternative health care delivery system. We recommend this information be provided in a provider manual or booklet.

It will be important for the physician and hospital personnel to get information relating to each plan or contracting company. The personnel in an outpatient setting who should receive this information are: the physician, physician office manager, any other physician office or medical group office personnel responsible for billing and posting of accounts receivable, and the receptionist. The personnel of the hospital who should receive this information include: hospital administration, including the administrator and associate or assistant administrators; business office manager and related personnel; hospital utilization review and quality assurance coordinators; patient advocates or patient representatives; admitting department personnel; and emergency room personnel.

The specific information disseminated to the provider should be very comprehensive and include all aspects of plan design and operation. In developing a specific format, the PPO may wish to consider different material for different providers (i.e., hospital or physician). Although material may be designed to be multi-functional for the sake of simplicity, this alternative may prove cumbersome and confusing.

The information should, at a minimum, include the following:

1. Level of reimbursement. Providers will be expected to accept the payment from the payor as payment in full. Business office and billing systems will require information relative to negotiated discount or rate so that the patient does not get billed.

2. Contracting payors of contracting companies. To assist providers in the verification process, it will be important to know which insurance companies and employers have entered into a PPO arrangement.

3. Means of eligibility verification. In order to ensure that the patient presenting himself for services is indeed covered so that the provider will be reimbursed for services provided, it is necessary to verify eligibility. Perhaps the most common approach is a local number for the provider to call, with appropriate access to this line. One of the causes of great concern in a PPO is the inability of a provider to verify patient eligibility, and the subsequent revelation that

the physician will have to look to the patient for payment rather than the contracting payor if the patient turns out to be ineligible.

4. Benefit coverages. It is important for the provider to know those services which are covered and those which are not in order to know whether to bill the patient's insurance company. Some PPO plans also have a co-insurance provision. If such is the case, the provider will also need to have this information. If the provider must call to verify eligibility, it is a good time to verify benefits and coverage, even if this information is already provided in some printed materials.

5. Procedural issues and internal operations. The providers must be made aware of the policies and procedures relating to each of the agreements entered into with an insurance company or employer. This may include such items as the format, criteria and requirements of the utilization review program, where to send bills for services rendered, handling of charges for lab tests done outside of the physicians office, and other reimbursement issues.

Employer issues

Upon selecting the PPO option, one of the major questions an employer will ask is, "How will this be marketed or presented to my employee?" This is a critical question because employee opinion begins to crystalize at this point.

Group meetings or group presentations are the best method of communicating the new concept. Literature given to the employee, without benefit of a meeting, is likely to be discarded. A group meeting affords PPO representatives the opportunity to answer any questions an employee might have. This form of interactive communication serves to enhance the utilization of preferred providers.

These meetings are an opportunity to explain how this alternative health care delivery system works and the specific benefits and drawbacks. It is an opportunity to explain how to use the health plan, keeping in mind that the PPO option may not be appropriate for all employees. This will also be a time to answer questions relating to price differentials in terms of employee contributions between the PPO plan and other plans being offered by the employer.

A payor-based PPO may be sensitive to the inclusion of providers in the marketing activities. However, to the extent that both parties see that inclusion as mutually beneficial, it will serve to meet the shared goal of enhanced utilization of designated providers.

Part of the education of subscribers should include a disclaimer regarding the number and type of physicians contracting to provide services within a PPO setting. It is unreasonable for a subscriber to believe that a PPO will be able to provide 100 per cent of the necessary care. Some physician networks may not have some super-specialized physicians, such as pediatric endocrinology, and subscribers should understand that this care is still available although outside the network on a different financial basis.

Claims processing

The role and ability of the PPO to process insurance claims is determined by the sponsorship of the PPO itself. For PPOs sponsored by third-party administrators or insurance carriers, one major activity is processing claims. These two organizations capture a major share of operating revenue from such claims processing. The vital issue addressed by such organizations is the ability to structure systems to process the "dual option" claim. For such claims, the system must be able to process and pay non-participating providers in a manner consistent with processing outside the PPO arrangement, while maintaining the ability to process claims for participating providers on an alternative fee arrangement. Although some claim systems have these capabilities today, most are in the process of development.

For provider-based PPOs, the issue of processing claims may have significant legal ramifications. In the state of California, provider-based PPOs that process claims may be required to meet the legal requirements of California Insurance Code 01 (the Knox-Keene Health Care Service Plan Act). This legislation was enacted to protect HMO subscribers from HMO failure. As such, when claims processing and providers are linked together through provider-based PPOs, the PPO may be required to comply with extensive regulations that are, for the most part, inapplicable and inappropriate for PPOs.

The ability of the provider-based PPO to process claims may, however, provide some competitive market advantage, since the PPO would have a broader base of functions. This competitive advantage, however, can be quickly eroded: providers have neither the market competence nor the proficiency to compete with firms that process claims for their livelihood.

For the provider-based PPO, it is important to clarify the claims processing. The processing organization must meet the payment methodology developed by the PPO. For example, if the PPO is structuring fixed physician-fee schedules and hospital per diem rates, the processing organization must have the systems capability to process claims under these types of fee structures.

How, and if, the PPO intervenes in the claims processing function to conduct medical or utilization review must also be examined. It is critical for PPOs to gather information pertaining to the services rendered by PPO providers because of the need to monitor efficiency. To that extent, it may be appropriate to establish a system whereby the PPO acts as the initial receiving point for this data collection prior to batching them and forwarding the claims on to the appropriate insurance payor. However, the PPO must be careful not to develop a competitive position in the marketplace with those entities with which it is seeking to do business. It appears that most insurance companies would be reluctant, at best, to relinquish their role as claims processor. If the provider based PPO seeks to process claims, it may find it extremely difficult to negotiate contracts with insurance companies or other payors who process claims.

Data needs and performance evaluation

Timely data reflecting the activity within the PPO is critical to PPO success. The PPO must be able to monitor and track the timeliness and appropriateness of payment from payors in order to evaluate payor performance. The PPO must also be able to track patient entrance into the system and evaluate the level of activity generated by each payor. Unless the PPO is capturing all claims data at one point in the process, the source for this data will likely be the PPO providers themselves. As such, the PPO providers—hospitals and physicians—must be able to track their financial source activity by specific payor.

Another need for data within the PPO system exists for the hospital itself. Hospitals participating in PPOs must have systems that allow them to analyze their specific per unit costs so they can intelligently price their services for reimbursement at a level consistent with financial viability.

Under the discount and per diem approaches to reimbursement, the hospital typically does not have the financial systems capability to access true costs. At present, it seems that those hospitals with the best ability to access true costs for intelligent pricing of PPO services, are those hospitals operating under some form of DRG methodology. A true cost accounting system must be developed to enable hospitals to evaluate costs and risks. These systems are currently being developed for government reimbursed programs and will lend themselves well to PPO arrangements.

A major component to the success or failure of the PPO will

be the effectiveness of physician members' medical practice habits. The utilization and practice habits of physicians within the PPO context is critical to the PPO's success. The development of these systems is currently underway in several organizations and may provide significant breakthroughs for "medical management" in the PPO arrangement. It should be noted that these systems are already in existence and use in HMOs.

For provider-based PPOs to maintain long-term effectiveness, it is suggested that they either develop relationships with contracting payors that enable them access to claims data to profile physicians' performance or develop independent systems to monitor and evaluate their physicians practice habits. Although the confidentiality of data collected through the PPO arrangement will principally fall under the purview of insurance legislation, it is necessary to consult with legal counsel to determine the extent and sensitivity of access to data. Issues of patient-provider relationships and medical review should also be considered within the legal review of data confidentiality.

Key elements to a successful PPO

Regardless of the type of PPO formed—be it payor, provider or entrepreneur based—certain ingredients dictate success. Generally, they fall into three categories: selecting the right providers, developing the appropriate incentives for providers and subscribers, and implementing the correct controls to ensure the ongoing viability of the organization.

With respect to provider selection, it is best to choose those hospitals and physicians that have demonstrated superior efficiency and effectiveness in the use of resources and medical practice. In this regard, insurance companies or large third-party administrators may have an advantage because of the utilization data at their disposal.

Providers must also be geographically well located to meet the needs of the subscribers of contracting entities. Obviously, it does little good to have a great network established if no one is going to use it. Also, the provider network should be constructed to insure the appropriate number of physicians and hospitals, including the appropriate mix of specialties and services. The providers within the PPO should provide high quality medical care, and the PPO should be able to point to established criteria or other data that can support this. Providers must be committed to making the PPO a success, for unless the providers feel they have a stake in the PPO—even in a payor based PPO— indifference may quickly lead to dissatisfaction which always is virtually impossible to hide from the subscriber. Hospitals and their medical staffs need to coordinate and work closely together for a variety of reasons, one of which has to do with the impact of per diem pricing on hospital reimbursement and the utilization of ancillary hospital services. Finally, the selection process should identify and screen out the inefficient and ineffective providers either prospectively or retrospectively. This is a very sensitive issue for a hospital administrator with respect to medical staff relations. Also, the PPO needs to be wary of violating any restraint of trade or other anti-trust laws.

The right incentives must be in place for both providers and subscribers in order to make a PPO program work. First, the providers need to be rewarded for efficient performance. This may take the form of either increased volume or rapid payment. It does a provider little good to participate in a PPO, frequently accepting less than 100 per cent as payment, if there is no *quid pro quo*.

Developing the right incentives may mean that providers go at risk. Payment may be based on guaranteed rates and include the per diem or DRG approaches, or may be more innovative such as a partial capitation or performance-based payment approach. In the last model, utilization goals could be set in advance (especially in the area of impatient utilization per 1,000 subscribers per year) and reimbursement could be based on how well the providers did in reaching that goal. Finally, the payment methodology adopted must take into consideration marketplace conditions, for the payor and provider alike. For example, hospital discounts offer no incentives for efficiency at any level. Unlike other approaches, discounting charges does not give the hospital any incentive to be efficient in the delivery of care. This also provides a reduced level of predictability for total expenses incurred by the insurance company.

In California, the Medicaid program is contracting with hospitals on an inclusive per diem basis (one specific amount per day regardless of the services rendered). Because of the price and cost sensitivity of this methodology, payors are quite favorably disposed to this development. With the implementation of reimbursement by diagnostic related groups (DRG) under the Medicare program, it is quite possible that this form of reimbursement may well become the state of the art for contracting with hospitals in a PPO setting. Because of the ease of administration, payors are looking to reimburse for physicians' services on a fixed-fee schedule, rather than a percentage of charges or a determination of usual, customary and reasonable rates. In summary, the rates of reimbursement must be competitive for providers and payors; providers must realize that reimbursement cannot be skewed to place the insurance company at risk; and, at the same time, the insurance company must realize that a certain level of payment is necessary to recruit and retain the physicians necessary to ensure a network that stresses and delivers quality medical care.

Developing the right controls essentially means the inclusion of the appropriate review mechanisms to eliminate unnecessary, unjustifiable services. Utilization review (UR) may take any one of three different forms: retrospective, concurrent or prospective. Some of the UR programs which a PPO may wish to adopt are:

1. Pre-admission review, to determine the need for medical care prior to admission to the hospital.

2. Admission certification, to determine the need for the patient to be admitted to an acute care hospital.

3. Continued stay review, to determine the need for the patient to continue his/her stay at the hospital.

4. Ancillary review, to determine the appropriateness and quality of ancillary services rendered.

5. Review of surgical necessity, to determine the appropriateness and quality of the surgical procedure performed.

It is important to keep in mind the relationship between the review programs and the payment method adopted. If the hospital is at risk for the quantity of ancillary services rendered under a per diem reimbursement arrangement, an ancillary review program may not be necessary. In any event, the decisions of the review process must ensure timely payment. The best interests of all participants is served if structures are in place to prevent unnecessary or otherwise inappropriate service. The right controls can be developed by ensuring the objectivity of the review process. Either PPO members or an independent external review organization—such as a professional services review organization—can be assigned responsibility for review activities. Or, the activity can be shared. Payors are skeptical of complete PPO control of utilization review because it smacks of self interest. On the other hand, providers may be reluctant to delegate total control to another party. Although the UR programs discussed here focus on inpatient care, there is no doubt that PPOs will begin to focus on outpatient care in the future, after demonstrating their ability to operate efficiently and effectively. Finally, although not mentioned explicitly, the successful PPO will require a quality assurance program to ensure the quality of services being rendered.

This discussion of operational issues is necessarily general. Each PPO will face its own problems, depending upon its structure and the specific functions it undertakes. Care in organizational development may indeed obviate these concerns as critical, operational issues.

CHAPTER NINE
Legal Issues

It can be argued that no area of law is changing any faster than is health care law. This change owes much of its impetus to the proliferation of new modes of delivery and the application of existing statutes to health care delivery via case law.

For the PPO, problems are compounded because there is no one, clearly accepted definition applicable to all PPOs and no statutory definition covers its provenance. Because the PPO develops its various forms as a pro-competitive strategy, the local marketplace has seved to particularize its characteristics: it is a concept, not a specific entity. Despite the lack of statutory definition—or perhaps even because of it—there is potential applicability of a broad variety of current statutory and case law to the PPO.

The primary areas of law that must be considered in relation to the preferred provider organization are:

- tax laws;

- federal anti-trust laws, including the Sherman Act, the FTC Act, the Clayton Act, the Robinson-Patman Act, and case law applied to these broad statutes as well as applicable state laws;

- securities, insurance and other health care coverage laws and regulations, both at the federal and state levels; and

- malpractice liability.

Tax laws and issues

Tax issues are primarily centered upon sponsorship of the PPO. Broadly speaking, PPOs are of three types: entrepreneurial (broker type), third-party payor-based, or provider-based. For either entrepreneurial or third-party payor-based PPOs, tax-exempt status may not be available, as these PPOs are analogous to profit-making businesses. If the PPO is run by profit-making entities, it is probably not tax-exempt, even if nonprofit. If the PPO is seen as primarily furthering commercial purposes, its ability to obtain tax-exempt status would be questionable. It should be noted in passing that IPAs no longer qualify for tax-exempt status.

A non-profit PPO organized and operated solely to benefit a

single, charitable hospital which is exempt under Internal Revenue Code §501(c)(3)—or a chain of related exempt hospitals—would most likely also be exempt. On the other hand, multiple-provider based PPOs appear to be ineligible for tax-exempt status under Internal Revenue Code §501(c)(3). A multi-provider PPO may not be classified under this category, because no charitable activity is carried on by the PPO and no services are rendered substantially below cost. The PPO may obtain a tax exemption under Internal Revenue Code §501(c)(4), as a "social welfare" organization, because some "community involvement" is present. However, many attorneys believe the applicability of this exemption remains unclear. If a PPO is organized and operated solely for private benefit of its participating providers it will not be tax-exempt. Many PPOs have, therefore, elected to operate as for-profit corporations.

Special tax considerations apply to the tax-exempt hospital participating in a PPO. The tax-exempt hospital may wish to carefully scrutinize the risk of PPO participation to its federal tax-exempt status. The issue of private inurement (because of expected benefits to private physicians and providers) violates tax-exemption laws and may apply if discounts are offered. This issue assumes importance only where physicians do not contribute their fair share of capital and operating costs (on the other hand it can be argued that the physicians' contractual obligations to the PPO are "sufficient consideration" for the hospital financing the PPO). Many in the industry, however, believe that prompt payment and increased volume may justify the risks.

To adequately protect the tax-exempt status of a non-profit hospital participating in a PPO, several firms specializing in PPO development have counseled hospital clients that care should be taken to continue support of community programs, to continue participation in the Medicare and Medicaid programs and to provide such services as emergency care to minimize risk to the hospital's tax-exempt status. Legal issues relevant to PPO organization formation are briefly covered in chapter 3.

Antitrust concerns

It is ironic that the PPO, created as a pro-competitive measure, should require extensive analysis and scrutiny under antitrust laws. Advocates of increased competition in health care have argued that PPOs promote competition by allowing organizations to negotiate price in their respective, local service areas, directly competing for the prized private pay patient market. Insurers have assumed that such alternative delivery systems as PPOs, because they are measures intended to increase competition and decrease or stabilize health care costs, would be encouraged as being in the public interest. Even the staff of the Federal Trade Commission has expressed "cautious optimism" that PPOs may be a pro-competitive element to slow the rise in health care costs. In a recent advisory opinion, the FTC approved the organization of a PPO proposed by Health Care Management Associates, a New Jersey consulting firm, as not violating federal antitrust laws.

Federal court decisions in the past few years have, however, shattered the illusion that health care "in the public interest" is exempt from antitrust laws. Supreme Court cases, such as *National Gerimedical Hospital and Gerontological Center v. Blue Cross of Kansas City* and *Arizona v. Maricopa County Medical Society,* have strongly, and with telling effect, applied antitrust laws to health care. It is clear that the PPO is subject to scrutiny for the legality of its program under applicable antitrust laws, and there is no doubt that potential antitrust exposure exists for providers participating in PPOs.

The four federal antitrust statutes that impinge upon PPO organization and operation include the Sherman Act, the Fair Trade Commission (FTC) Act, the Clayton Act and the Robinson-Patman amendment to the Clayton Act.

The Sherman Act, Section 1, prohibits contracts, combinations and conspiracies in restraint of trade. Any activity, discussion or agreement between competing providers concerning price, division of market, allocation of service or territories or exclusive dealing between providers and purchasers is subject to scrutiny as anti-competitive action. Section 2 of the Sherman Act discusses and prohibits monopolization, attempts to monopolize and conspiracies to monopolize.

Civil or criminal liability can ensue from violations of both sections of the Sherman Act. Treble damages may be assessed for proven violations of the Sherman Act in suits by private parties. Civil and criminal government enforcement of the statute lies with the Department of Justice. The FTC Act prohibits unfair methods of competition and unfair or deceptive acts or practices (Section 5). This consumer protection statute encompasses violations of both the Sherman and Clayton acts. The Federal Trade Commission is responsible for enforcement of this Act. The Clayton Act and its amendment, the Robinson-Patman Act, deal primarily with goods and may be applicable in the formation of hospital joint ventures and unlawful mergers.

In dealing with anti-trust issues, the courts have used two tests to analyze allegations: (1) the "rule of reason" test and (2) *per se* violation test. The "rule of reason" test is a factual analysis decided on a case-by-case basis. The court reviews the activities and agreements which restrain trade and then analyzes the nature, purpose and effect of the restraint. The court must determine, through its analysis, whether the alleged violation fits within the range of legitimate business efforts and promotes competitive rivalry or whether its primary trust (and effect) is anti-competitive. The courts, in practice, have not found an anti-trust violation when the practice which restrains trade is reasonable in light of its nature, purpose and effect. A reasonable level of restraint is, therefore, not a violation of antitrust law given a strong business and efficiency justification.

There are, however, certain practices that the courts have always found to be anti-competitive. These are called *per se* violations. A *per se* violation results in what attorneys call a "conclusive presumption" that the practices are illegal. If a *per se* violation exists, no "rule of reason" test is made. The practice is automatically found to be an antitrust violation, and the defendant is prohibited from submitting pro-competitive justifications for consideration at the trial. By contrast, when the "rule of reason" test is applied, extensive inquiry is made into the pro-competitive aspects of the alleged violation.

Per se violations include (1) "horizontal price fixing," or agreements among competitors to affect prices; (2) "horizontal market divisions," or agreements to divide service or geographic markets; and (3) "horizontal boycotts," or refusal to deal with others. *Per se* violations could result in liability for substantial civil damages and criminal penalties. Additionally, the financial and individual burdens of defending against an antitrust action are usually substantial.

Broad as the federal statutes are, it is specific case law that determines applicability of antitrust principles to the PPO. Within a defined service area, independent hospitals are considered competitors under antitrust laws. Similarly, physician practice entities—whether individuals, partnerships or incorporated medical practices in the same defined service area—are also deemed competitors. It should be noted, however, that the definition of the relevant service area, as well as the determination of whether the defendant entity is affecting interstate commerce, must be decided on a case-by-case basis.

In 1981, the U.S. Supreme Court ruled on a major issue: whether there was an implied repeal of antitrust laws by subsequently enacted legislation in the health care field. The Court ruled (*National Gerimedical Hospital and Gerontology Center v. Blue Cross of Kansas City*, 452 U.S. 378 [1981]) that the federal health planning legislation of 1974, P.L. 93-641, did not by implication repeal the Sherman Act. The ruling reconfirmed that the health care field, despite its prior assumption to the contrary, was subject to the same antitrust laws as all businesses.

In this case, the Blue Cross Plan presumed that P.L. 93-641

would, in the interest of efficient distribution of health care facilities, encourage the division of the local market by existing health care providers. The Blue Cross Plan therefore refused to contract with a new investor-owned hospital because the hospital's construction had not been approved by the local Health Systems Agency (HSA). The hospital brought suit, predicating violation of the Sherman Act based upon alleged conspiracy between the planning agency and the Blue Cross Plan. It was, the hospital claimed, a conspiracy in restraint of trade and competition.

The Supreme Court ruled that it was not the intent of Congress to lift the application of antitrust laws in order to carry out the hospital facility planning process. The court ruled that the HSA, although created by federal law and financed by federal funds, was only advisory and not regulatory. It was, therefore, a private party like Blue Cross. These private parties could not compel restrictions in the name of carrying out governmental programs. The court further explained that only an official government agency could compel or arrange hospital mergers and restrictions on competition without resultant antitrust scrutiny.

If the *National Gerimedical Hospital and Gerontological Center v. Blue Cross of Kansas City* case firmly placed health care within the context of antitrust purview, then the *Maricopa* decision focused antitrust scrutiny directly upon the PPO itself.

In 1982, the Supreme Court eliminated the ''presumed benefit of the doubt'' thought applicable to concerted action in the health care field (*Arizona v. Maricopa County Medical Society*, 73 L. Ed. 2d 48 [1982]). Some 70 per cent of the physicians in Maricopa County, to counteract HMOs and other competition, organized the Tucson and Phoenix Foundation as a nonprofit organization. This foundation for medical care functioned essentially as a physician-based PPO and utilized a ''maximum fee'' schedule approved by majority vote of the organization. The agreement to accept a maximum fee schedule on behalf of certain insured patients was binding on all participants.

It was thought that the "rule of reason" test would be applied to allow this practice as a reasonable restraint of trade, as the foundation's "maximum fee" schedule was in the interest of more cost-efficient patient care. This concept is, however, diametrically opposed to the concept that price-fixing by competitors is a *per se* actionable antitrust violation. The state filed suit, claiming that the maximum fee schedules were nothing more than price-fixing by would-be competitors.

The Court held that the fee schedules, although purporting to set "maximum," not "minimum," fees, simply fixed fees. The fee schedules therefore rewarded skilled and unskilled practitioners alike, thereby discouraging fee competition, innovation in treatment, and the entry of new physicians to the area. The Court further found that such "maximum fees" constituted conventional horizontal price fixing, which is a *per se* violation of Section 1 of the Sherman Act. Consequently, the Court refused to consider asserted pro-competition and cost reducing effects, giving no special consideration because health care professionals were involved.

Although the *Maricopa* decision found the establishment of a fee schedule by the physician-controlled PPO to be illegal, the Court was careful to limit its decision: "it is not necessary," the decision read, "that the doctors do the price fixing." The ruling further noted that an insurer may fix the fee schedule and enter into bilateral contracts with individual doctors. (The Department of Justice has previously expressed the opinion in *Group Life & Health Insurance Company v. Royal Drug Company,* that such an arrangement would be legal unless plaintiffs could establish that a conspiracy among providers was at work.)

In the *Maricopa* case, the antitrust problems arose because competitors reached an agreement on prices to be paid by certain insurers. Illegal price fixing would also be found if a group of hospitals (like the physicians) were to agree upon prices to be charged to third-party payors.

In contrast, an independent, nonprovider-controlled PPO administrator might, consistent with the *Maricopa* decision and the Sherman Act, establish a fee schedule and contract with participating providers as the agent of insurers or employer groups. It is generally permissible for a third-party payor to establish a uniform rate. However, even if the third-party payor were to insist upon the establishment of uniform prices or discounts by hospitals and physicians, jointly participating in the PPO, the payor would not necessarily be precluded from later pursuing antitrust action against the providers.

Where uniform prices (or discounts) are fixed by a PPO—owned or controlled by hospitals or other providers—antitrust issues will surely arise, unless the organizers are offering a new form of health care delivery system. There is no price fixing if the PPO is a joint venture construed as a "single economic unit" within the framework of antitrust laws. In general, joint ventures survive antitrust scrutiny because of the principle that a single entity is incapable of conspiring against itself.

It must be noted, however, that the formation of joint ventures among otherwise unrelated hospitals will result in antitrust liability, if the joint venture is merely a vehicle for price-fixing among competitors already operating in the marketplace. The hospitals must form a distinct economic unit, through merger or an affiliation under a common parent holding company, sharing financial risks and revenue. In the *Maricopa* case, the Court noted

> . . . The foundations are not analogous to partnerships or other joint arrangements in which persons who would otherwise be competitors pool their capital and share the risks of loss as well as the opportunities for profit. In such joint ventures, the partnership is regarded as a single firm competing with other sellers in the market.

Three additional issues must be considered in the formation of a joint venture by hospitals and physicians:

1. whether the formation of the joint venture presents a "merger" problem under antitrust law;

2. whether the purpose of the joint venture is lawful; and

3. whether the agreements entered into by participants are necessary to carry out the joint venture's activities.

Merger and monopolization issues are immediately raised if a substantial percentage of providers within a service area participate in a joint venture. The U.S. Supreme Court held, in the *United States v. Penn-Olin Chemical Company,* 378 U.S. 158 (1964), that joint ventures must be analyzed under Section 7 of the Clayton Antitrust Act to determine anti-competitive effect. That section declares unlawful any merger that creates a monopoly in any market or that substantially lessens competition. (Other mergers would be subject to similar analyses under Sections One and Two of the Sherman Act.)

It has been suggested (by the Hospital Council of Southern California: *Preferred Provider Organization Contracting Manual,* 1983) that an enterprise which accounts for less than 15 per cent of a service market is not likely to found in violation of antitrust prohibitions. It has also been suggested by the same source that 40 per cent combined market share may be used as a benchmark for "substantial" market share sufficient to raise antitrust violation concerns.

In *United States v. Sealy, Inc.,* 388 U.S. 350 (1973), the Court found that if the purpose of the joint venture is merely to allow competing businesses to enter into an otherwise unlawful act, the joint venture itself will be found unlawful. If, however, economic justification exists for a joint venture—for example, where the participants are unable to produce the service or product of the joint venture without association—the joint ventures have been held to be lawful. And, as in the *Maricopa* decision, a joint venture among health care providers is permissible if participants "pool their capital and share the risk of loss as well as the opportunities for profit."

The legality of a joint venture will not, however, legalize restraint on competition resulting from agreements among the participants. The Court in *Maricopa* cited its 1940 decision in *U.S. v. Socony-Vacuum Oil Company:*

> ... any combination that tampers with price structures is engaged in unlawful activity. Even though the members of the price-fixing group were in no position to control the market, to the extent they raised, lowered or stabilized prices, they would be directly interfering with the free play of market forces.

Several antitrust lawsuits have been filed on another issue: unlawful exclusion or boycott. In the case of *Hahn v. Oregon Physicians Service,* CA No. 81 3173, U.S. Court of Appeals (9th circuit), October 5, 1982, podiatrists filed suit against several prepaid health plans. Because the case challenged the right of HMOs and health benefit programs to exclude podiatrists as a class from the provision of services, the principal issue may be applicable to the PPO. Within the benefit schedules established for providers, classes of physicians may file suit and assert that they have an alleged right to provide services to the PPO client base.

A possible allegation could be made that the PPO has, in effect, combined with payors and participating providers (hospitals and physicians) to exclude a class of providers. The PPO could, however, reply that the requirement that participating physicians and other practitioners maintain membership on participating hospitals' medical staffs and the schedule of payors' benefits have denied discretion to the PPO by limiting expansion of the range of providers.

An allied issue which may be applicable to the PPO is "concerted refusals to deal." The Federal Trade Commission found that a group of dentists acted illegally in concert by agreeing to refuse dental insurance plans access to radiological films for utilization review. This agreement between separate members not to deal with a payor or to restrict the terms of dealing may constitute an illegal boycott under antitrust statutes. In this case, the FTC so found (See *In re Indiana Federation of Dentists,* FTC Docket No. 9118, February 18, 1983.) This case may have applicable implications for PPO participants.

Antitrust problems are not limited to provider actions. Third-party payors, including Blue Cross, Blue Shield and commercial health insurers may be challenged on the use of peer review committees, if these committees are used to determine if charged fees are reasonable or services rendered are needed. In *Union Labor Life Insurance Company v. Pireno,* 73L. Ed. 2d 647 (1982), the allegation was a conspiracy to eliminate price differences among practitioners, thereby violating Section 1 of the Sherman Act. The insurance company and the professional association of chiropractors that did peer review were alleged to conspire to fix the prices chiropractors would be allowed to charge.

Under the McCarran-Ferguson Act, most activities of insurance carriers are exempt from federal antitrust jurisdiction, if such activities are state regulated. This defense was raised in this case, but with little success. The Court held that the antitrust exemption applied only to the ''business of insurance''; that the use of a peer review committee by an insurer is not an integral part of the business of insurance, and that such use of peer review was, therefore, not exempt from antitrust scrutiny.

The case has important implications for utilization review and concurrent review programs by PPOs. No review program will be exempt from antitrust scrutiny solely because it is done on behalf of insurance companies and therefore presumed exempt. That presumption has been effectively shattered.

No discussion of antitrust issues can fail to discuss litigation and motivations. Competing providers excluded from participation in the PPO, whose markets have been reduced, may well sue.

Third-party payors may be impelled to sue by asserting damage to business through horizontal price fixing conspiracies or illegal boycotts. Where found, antitrust violations include liability for treble damages, punitive damage and recovery of legal fees.

The consumer, too, has what is called "a cause of action in antitrust law." Where an objectionable exclusion prevents a patient from being treated by the kind of practitioner he or she preferred, that patient may sue for damages. In *Blue Shield v. Virginia v. McCready,* 73L. Ed. 2d 149 (1982), the U.S. Supreme Court ruled that consumers of health services are the parties to be protected against selective refusal to reimburse—an anti-competitive practice. Should insured patients be able to prove that they have suffered financial injury, treble damages may be awarded.

It is unfortunate, but true, that federal antitrust statutes are not the only considerations. PPOs are subject to a broad range of antitrust laws promulgated by the respective states. Participants in PPO activities are advised to consult legal counsel for state antitrust statutes applicable to their programs, including the relevance of state laws on illegal trusts and insurance laws.

What guidelines may generally be used in PPO formation to obviate antitrust problems? The following points are offered for consideration:

- Provider-controlled PPO participants should avoid discussions and agreements concerning fees or uniform discount rates or agreement concerning allocation of services or territories. These agreements would constitute *per se* violations of antitrust laws.

- Formation of a joint venture PPO through a combination of hospitals is not advisable if it confers substantial competitive advantage or it substantially lessens competition in a given geographical market.

- If a joint venture PPO is formed, legal counsel should carefully review manner and method of contract negotiation prior to implementation. Legal counsel should also undertake merger analysis under Section 7 of the Clayton Act and use Department of Justice Merger Guidelines.

- The joint venture should be subject to lawful purpose analysis, including examination of economic justification and the pooling of capital and risk sharing.

- Physician arrangements should also be carefully examined, with FTC guidelines used for merger analysis (Federal Trade Commission Statement of Enforcement Policy, 46 Fed. Reg. 1982, at 48982, October 5, 1981). Anti-competitive conduct, especially with regard to the *Maricopa* decision, should be stringently examined. Should one or more physician groups participate in the ownership and control of the PPO, the same antitrust issues regarding contracting with hospitals will arise.

Although serious antitrust issues surround the formation and operation of preferred provider organizations, the consensus is that these are not insurmountable. Potential participants are urged to give thoughtful evaluation to risks before proceeding, to minimize the severity of the antitrust problems.

Insurance laws and regulations

The general thrust of health insurance regulations has traditionally been to insure purchasers of coverage protection from the risk of third-party failure, as well as guaranteed access to adequate health services. Insurance laws and regulations are targeted to see that:

1. financial risks are met through reasonable reserves for indemnity by the regulated entity;

2. reasonable value is provided to the consumer, through stringent regulation of the form and content of provider-subscriber agreements.

The focal point of such protective regulation has been the consumer. Protection of provider interests is not the major focus of regulatory intervention.

With respect to the PPO, a significant issue is whether the PPO is subject to regulation and/or state licensure—either as an indemnity plan or as a health maintenance organization (HMO). The current wisdom holds that significant loopholes in the statutes and regulatory requirements of most states allow operation of nonregulated systems, such as the PPO.

Depending upon the circumstances of its organization and administration and its geographic locale, the PPO may be subject to qualification and/or licensure under state and federal securities laws and under state insurance or prepaid health plan laws and regulations. If participants in the PPO are required to make a financial contribution in the form of membership fees, dues, or assessments, securities laws may apply. If the organization is "at risk" in any way, compliance with insurance or prepaid health plan laws and regulations may also be required.

In California, for example, provision of health care benefits are covered under three statutes and their regulations:

1. California Insurance Code regarding indemnity insurers;

2. Nonprofit Hospital Service Plans Act covering plans such as Blue Cross/Blue Shield;

3. Knox-Keene Health Care Service Plan Act, governing HMOs.

With the passage of A.B. 3480, in 1982, insurance companies are now allowed to discriminate between providers, by entering into "preferred provider" agreements. Many experts believe that PPOs in California are not governed under Insurance laws or the Service Plans Act. Neither, they contend, can the PPO with its delivery system or payment arrangements, be construed to be compatible with the health maintenance organization structure and therefore, it cannot be regulated as such under the

Knox-Keene Act. The PPO appears to be merely an administrative and marketing construct, not an insurance plan or HMO.

Those contemplating organizing PPOs should, however, be cautioned that legal counsel should thoroughly research applicable state statutes and regulations in their respective jurisdictions. PPOs undertake several of the functions of both indemnity plans and HMOs. For example, they arguably undertake to "arrange for" the provision of health benefits and some PPOs also incorporate claims processing and administrative services like indemnity plans. It is local state law and local state regulation that determines whether a PPO is feasible and/or governed by regulatory and licensure requirements.

ERISA

Where PPOs provide services to employer self-insured or self-funded employee benefits plans, application of state law may be avoided. The Federal Employee Income Retirement Security Act of 1975 (ERISA) regulates employee pension plans, as well as employee welfare plans, including health coverage. The significance of the inclusion of health coverages rests with a clause pre-empting state regulation of all pension and welfare benefits under the terms of the Act. Thus, employee benefit plans operated directly by individual employers, unions or certain trust arrangements are exempt from application of state insurance or prepaid health plan regulation. These plans are outside the scope of state review by virtue of ERISA pre-emption. However, the ERISA pre-emption was substantially limited this year by an amendment to the Act. The amendment defines "multiple employer welfare arrangements" (MEWAs) as employee welfare benefit plans operated on behalf of more than one employer and states that such MEWAs are not exempt from state law. Thus, the possibility of a PPO receiving protection from application of state law by serving ERISA plans is limited by this recent amendment to the Act.

It has been hypothesized that to the extent PPOs serve employer welfare benefit plans as "administrative structures," PPOs could claim exemption under ERISA. However, a PPO, if involved in the management of an ERISA plan or in the disposition of ERISA plan assets, could be found to have fiduciary responsibilities and therefore fiduciary status under the Act, with all its liabilities. These points, are, however, untested and must await clarification by case law.

Malpractice concerns

Initially, the so-called PPO arrangements were simple, dual-choice arrangements offered by self-insured multi-employer trusts, under which the trust negotiated a discount from current retail charges from its preferred providers, whether physicians or hospitals, in consideration for listing them on the trust's provider panel. If the insured went to the preferred provider, then the insured were to get either full coverage or at least better coverage than if they went to a non-panel provider. Such arrangements, in themselves, do not appear to have any identified malpractice problems, as each provider—whether physician or hospital—is an independent contractor and is solely responsible for its own acts, and the patient has a free choice of provider.

However, the PPO arrangements have become much more sophisticated and structured. Providers now group into organizational structures, such as professional corporations, partnerships, joint ventures and trusts. Potentially there can be joint and several liability for all participants. Since the participant may be insured with different carriers with different limits as well as varying policy terms, the inter-party relationship in the event of a malpractice claim can be confusing, particularly if one or more of the parties is initially uninsured or underinsured. If the employer or the third-party purchaser of the PPO services requires an indemnity provision, the hospital or physician executing such a provision may find that its insurance policy specifically excludes coverage for liability assumed under an indemnity agreement. In effect, there is no insurance to cover the liability created by the indemnity provision.

The solution is provision of a wrap-around policy to cover overall exposure. These policies are not cheap, and the cost is substantially set by the extent of the underlying coverage of individual participants. There also remains the issue of coverage for claims of anti-trust activities of the PPO.

There are, also, special problems created by the PPO operation itself. So long as the PPO relied on discounts as the base of cost savings, there were few unique problems. However, it is now clear that to be cost effective, the PPO must increasingly rely on a strict utilization review program. It is through the faulty implementation of such programs that there can be potentially critical malpractice problems or factors that will aggravate an existing problem.

The first issue within the context of utilization review is the matter of pre-admission certification. If the patient believes that he or she has been denied needed treatment because of the denial of pre-admission certification of benefits by the utilization review program, then the patient may initiate legal action for damage from all participants in the process. If the pre-admission certification is performed by an outside entity, the exposure of the hospital itself may be minimal. However, the patient's physician may be found to be negligent, if he or she has not adequately presented the facts or the necessity of admission to the party performing the pre-admission certification. The difficult question facing both the physician and the hospital is whether or not to admit the patient regardless of the decision of the utilization review entity and to take the financial risk as to ultimate payment for service.

Usually, some type of structured appeal procedure is available, which should be diligently pursued if conditions warrant. It is important that all parties properly document the facts and the process followed to protect themselves if they are second guessed by a lawsuit in the event of an adverse result. If the denial is decreed to be arbitrary or capricious, there is potential for the award of punitive damages. This is a newly developing area of law in which the courts will be required to judge public policy of cost control versus the duty to provide all necessary care. Juries and the courts, it is anticipated, will find for the injured patient. "Obviously," states James E. Ludlam of Musick, Peeler and Garrett, "if the patient is provided with appropriate out-patient care, the liability exposure will be minimized."

The second and more complex issue relates to conflicts arising out of concurrent review procedures. Here we have an outside force, either within the hospital structure or imposed from the outside by the third-party payor, that will be making judgments on the matter of "medical necessity." These judgments conflict with those of the attending physician. Although the decision may only have the direct impact of determining whether or not there will be a third-party payment for the extended stay or for the proposed medical or surgical procedures proposed to be followed, the effect on the patient (directly or indirectly) is to either terminate the stay or provide that such extended stay—at demand of the patient—must be paid for at the patient's own expense. In such an event, a patient may elect to forgo what is later determined to be necessary treatment, with a serious adverse result. Historically, this decision was decided, if at all, in the context of a retroactive denial of coverage after the patient had received the care. The situation of deciding to treat or not to treat in advance is much more explosive.

Legally, the parties have conflicting responsibilities. Several issues can be clearly identified at this time in the evolution of the definition of the legal problems:

1. The competence of the utilization review personnel to make a judgement. This includes not only the screening personnel but also the person making the ultimate judgment of denial.

2. The process itself and particularly the degree to which the matter is investigated and the appellate process applied. This, of course, includes such important elements as the consultation with the attending physician and access to the current medical records, among other factors.

3. The problem of communication with the patient. This is a complex issue which starts from the point of purchase or receipt of coverage. Does the insured know of the limitation on his or her rights and those of the attending physician resulting from the UR process? In the event that the extension of the length of stay or the care is not approved by the review entity, who communicates the decision to the patient or the patient's representative, and even more important, what is communicated to the patient? Is the patient given the clear option to follow his own physician's judgment and,—if so, what penalty—or what pressure real or apparent—is put on the patient to accept discharge or denial of treatments.

Again, this is a relatively new area of potential liability. At this point, we do have the example of one trial court case involving a suit against a Medi-Cal utilization reviewer who denied an extension of stay. The patient claimed serious complications resulted. The jury granted a judgment of $500,000 against the state and the reviewer. Of interest is that the patient did not sue her physician who permitted her to be discharged—she felt he was also a victim of the system. This case, however, involved the problem of the competence of the UR reviewer, the process itself, and highlights the potential responsibility of the attending physician and the hospital. James E. Ludlam offers the opinion that if the patient had pressed an action against the physician and the hospital, there would have been a strong probability of their being held jointly liable with the UR entity. In other words, both the hospital and the physician have an independent duty of care to the patient, regardless of the action by the review entity.

To a substantial extent, these are problems and relationships that are faced routinely in the interplay between patients' health care providers and third-party payors: this may be a matter of an increased degree of liability exposure.

One interesting manifestation of the recognition of the implication of these relationships is the attempt by the various parties involved to shift the liability from one party to another through the use of indemnity agreements. Any party requested to indemnify another must be exceedingly careful to understand the legal impact of such action. It is one thing to indemnify against one's own conduct, but to assume responsibility for the conduct of another is quite different. Also, in the context of insurance, a liability assumed through an indemnity contract may not be covered by the liability insurance policy. To the extent then that the third party payor or its utilization review entity seeks to be included as an additional insured under the physician or the hospital's policy, there is an even more critical problem—not only the availability of such coverage but also its cost.

Regardless of the legal problems involved in utilization review, it is here to stay. The challenge to both physicians and hospitals is to make it work in the ultimate best interest of monitoring both cost and quality of care to the patient.

This leads to the question of whether UR should be performed on a delegated basis or whether it should be performed by an outside, independent entity. Currently, this is a highly controversial issue. From the viewpoint of potential liability problems and the more effective participation of the patient's personal physician, experience indicates that the delegated review is most protective of potential liability problems. On the other hand, there is always the question of the effectiveness of the process. For this reason, with the delegated review, there must be effective monitoring mechanisms to ensure accountability.

CHAPTER TEN

Evaluating the PPO Alternative

*Lessons and projections from operating PPOs—
including experiences from the PPO plan serving
employees of the Lutheran Hospital Society of
Southern California since 1975.*

The PPO, in concept and practice, can only be evaluated within the context of the dramatic changes that are occurring in the health care field. The transitions underway at this time influence the cost, reimbursement and organization of health care delivery. New programs, new services and the implementation of diverse management techniques (among them the PPO) have evolved to meet the challenges posed by transition to a more competitive health care marketplace.

The widespread interest the concept has created—and the subsequent proliferation of PPOs in various permutations—make evaluation a difficult task, although developments appear promising. Versions of preferred provider organizations have obviously been in existence for some time and have proven to be viable. The existing models, however, have typically operated in controlled environments. That is, the contracted provider and the contracted payer have some form of organizational linkage. An example, of course, is our own preferred provider organization that has served the employees of the Lutheran Hospital Society of Southern California (LHS) since 1975. The society has contracted with hospitals and doctors and developed a benefit package whereby employees have a significant financial incentive to utilize participating providers.

Success, in terms of cost control and employee utilization within the provider network, can be measured. Independent study has demonstrated that LHS's PPO has produced savings when measured against experience in comparable populations. Furthermore, there has been a distinct shift in utilization patterns from outside providers to those within the network, during the time of the PPO's operation. It has been demonstrated that cost savings totalled between $300,000 to $400,000 for each year of operation for LHS's PPO. But many question the portability of this success pattern to other PPOs, particularly in addressing the open, uncontrolled market. In addition, as PPOs begin to experiment with various designs, it becomes much more difficult to prognosticate the potential for success for all of the options.

Potential for success

As a concept, the PPO alternative has enormous appeal: it has something for everyone. The claim has been made that "PPO formation can offer many benefits to all of the parties at interest in the health-care market."[1] The widest claims have been made for benefits to accrue to hospital providers. From the point of view of the payer, or sponsoring entity, the measure of a PPO's success over time would be its ability to hold down or restrain the rate of growth in the health care costs borne by the group. From the point of view of the provider, the measure of success will be indicated by an increase in utilization and business volume and an improvement in the payor mix. That is, more of the participants in the provider service will be sponsored by groups who do, in fact, pay assured prices.

PPOs have, it is claimed, the potential for helping hospitals sustain an adequate patient base, competitively positioning the hospital in the marketplace. The claim is further made that PPOs can broaden the hospitals' patient base by admitting more physicians to the medical staff and creating outpatient service demands by the increased patient pool. The possibilities foreseen for the PPO concept are limitless, including the creation of a continuum of care: from wellness, occupational safety and health programs, employee counseling, acute care, long-term care and consultation services to employers.

In Denver, the PPO experience is reportedly positive: three PPOs accomplished this cost savings (of approximately 20 per cent to insurers) through negotiating discounts between providers and insurers, eliminating unnecessary red tape and streamlining administrative procedures, controlling usual and customary charges, involving employers directly with health care providers and educating PPO plan participants.[2] Hospital charges were typically discounted 7 per cent.[3] Despite the discounts, the Denver experience is claimed to offer improved cash flow to providers and the reduction of bad debts to minimal levels, while creating a greater patient base.

For physicians, the PPO is seen as preserving the traditional doctor-patient relationship, as well as fee-for-service payment. Participation in PPOs is also seen as lessening the threat of closed hospital medical staffs. With an overabundance of physicians in many areas, and the supply of physicians estimated to increase by 43 per cent over the period from 1978 to 1990, the PPO assumes greater importance as a means of maintaining a viable private practice.[4]

Attractive as the PPO concept may be, in practice the PPO can work to negative advantage through discounting fees. Denver area PPOs offer 7–30 per cent discounts on the fees of more than 500 physician participants in three plans.[5]

The PPO has important implications for modifying physician behaviors, as well as offering a competitive advantage. Many PPOs are looking to the establishment of utilization review mechanisms—including extensive data collection and analysis—to provide physicians with feedback, so that unnecessary inpatient care is eliminated. The feedback mechanisms will, hopefully, ensure the provision of all necessary services at appropriate levels of care, while aiding physicians in self-monitoring for cost containment and peer review activities. The PPO concept incorporates, in all its permutations, the principle of physician accountability. This evaluation is crucial to operational success. Developing PPOs need to ensure the availability of this type of data.

The consumer of health care services also realizes real benefits from the PPO. It guarantees freedom of choice, unlike the HMO model which sharply restricts consumer options. It typically offers financial incentives to use a preferred provider, although it offers the consumer the option of using other providers at additional cost.

It could be reasonably argued that the most appropriate measure of success would be the acceptance of the PPO and of its services by the subscribing public. Public marketplace satisfaction, however, is several removes from the decisions which affect implementation and practice.

As this book notes, although the concept of the PPO represents an elegant simplicity, the translation of concept into organized practice requires integration. First of all, the payer and provider have to agree to contract for services on a PPO basis. Then the payer, or sponsoring insurance company, has to offer the program to an employer or other sponsored group. Next, the sponsored group or employer has to offer the PPO as an alternative to the existing health payment mechanisms, including general insurance programs and HMOs. Once employees or subscribers elect to participate in the PPO, they then have a choice at the time that they need services. If the incentives, both financial and qualitative (relative to the reputation or accessibility of the provider) are sufficient, then the employees or subscriber will elect to utilize the provider network. In effect, five decisions have to be made before a service is rendered to a consumer under the PPO umbrella.

Just as the PPO is an attractive alternative for consumers because of financial incentives, negotiated rates and controls through utilization review are the attractions for employer groups and insurers. Negotiated rates through the PPO represent predictability of health care costs and, in some instances, realizable savings. Given the sharp increases in health care costs over the past few years, predictability assumes increased importance to insurers and employers, because premium rate increases are historical adjustments.

During the past year, benefit cuts and upward price adjustments in premiums, often by 25 per cent or more, were undertaken by many Blue Cross/Blue Shield plans and commercial insurance companies. Part of the problem was an 18.7 per cent increase in hospital costs in 1981.[6] The prognosis for 1983 groups health insurance rates remain grim. Insurers are predicting average rate hikes of 25–35 per cent.[7] The "culprits," besides inflation, are seen as increased utilization and cost-shifting. Transamerica Occidental epitomizes the plight and performance of group health insurers: it announced a pretax loss of $56 million for the third quarter of 1982.[8]

As premiums escalate, health care costs have come to dominate the concerns expressed by benefits managers. In 1982, a survey of the Fortune 100 benefits managers done by Martin E. Segal Company reported that nearly 50 per cent of those managers listed medical cost containment as their number one concern.[9] By contrast, only 4 per cent thought health care cost was their biggest problem in 1978. At the current rate of growth, it has been estimated that health care costs will total $462.2 billion in 1985. In 1990, the estimated costs will run to $821 billion. (See exhibit 1.4, chapter 1.)

Employers have, over time, become more sophisticated in their approaches. Discounts and negotiated rates represent the current and necessary first step. The long-range implications have assumed increased importance. Cost control is no longer a stop-gap measure: it is strategic, corporate selection through realization of buying power. Employers are aware, as never before, that they may direct their employees to providers with certain styles of practice. Selectivity is now the name of the game for cost effectiveness, as employers integrate various approaches to health care costs through their own initiatives. Coalitions and alliances have been created within the past few years to build data bases and marshall the resources necessary for concerted attention. As employers decide that they have a major stake in the outcome and flex their economic power, the impact of their decisions will have major repercussions on current and anticipated practice styles and systems.

The rise in costs have assumed importance not only in the private sector, they have come to dominate public policy discussion as well. John K. Iglehart's "Health Policy Report," in the *New England Journal of Medicine,* January 27, 1983, notes that[10]

. . . absent from the [Reagan] administration's list of accomplishment is the enactment of legislation to implement its belief that marketplace principles should be relied on to moderate costs and increase efficiency in health care . . . the administration has not yet backed its rhetoric with a legislative proposal. But in this instance, legislative steps have been taken at the federal and state levels that suggest that price competition in medical care is intensifying, even without a concerted drive by the Reagan administration.

Less dependence on Washington's "largesse" is anticipated, with state and local governments, private corporate buyers of medical care and providers—including hospitals and physicians —evaluating their own priorities and charting their own courses for future survival. The PPO is seen as one viable alternative.

The consensus of informed opinion contends that there is a clear pattern which explains the impetus for PPO development: a respnse of traditional health providers to increased competition in the local market. This is confirmed by a survey conducted by the California Hospital Association.[11] Those who responded to the survey overwhelmingly gave market share responses.

What were your primary reasons for joining or forming a PPO?

- 95 per cent, to protect or increase current market share;

- 88 per cent, to protect or increase occupancy rates;

- 54 per cent, in response to local market place demand;

- 29 per cent, in response to cost shifting anticipated as a result of Medi-Cal negotiations;

- 24 per cent, in response to requests from the medical staff; and

- 20 per cent, in response to encroachment by Health Maintenance Organizations.

PPOs as a competitive edge

It seems clear, then, that PPOs are overwhelmingly seen as a competitive edge: California hospitals see PPOs as offering a competitive advantage against other hospitals and against HMOs. Physicians, too, often raise the issue of competitive advantage, particularly with respect to advantage against hospitals via discounts for services in outpatient settings.

Given an increasingly competitive environment, given a concept that promises so much to so many, how have PPOs performed? If growth is an index of performance, the PPO has been phenomenally successful. According to all reports, the most intensive PPO growth has centered in California:[12]

> Of those 286 hospitals, 11 per cent already contract with a PPO, 22 per cent are forming a PPO, and 39 per cent are interested in doing so.

The AHA Center for Multi-Institutional Arrangements notes that the phenomenon is not limited to California. Operational PPOs now exist in thirteen states. A survey taken in September 1982 (sponsored by HealthWest Foundation and conducted by the AHA Center for Multi-Institutional Arrangements) found that 84 hospitals participated in PPOs at the time, with 700 more considering participation.[13]

Where the problems lie

Despite the claimed successes, several caveats must be raised. The proliferation of PPOs could result in patient shuffling between providers, without increase in market share for any provider. It has been noted that despite the escalations in cost of care, the total market for health care is not growing.[14] Many astute observers of the health care scene note that the frenzied interest in PPOs may be reactionary, attributable to the fear that unless the provider affiliates with a PPO, other affiliated providers may steal their private-pay patient base.

It could be argued, of course, that what providers are seeking is not merely to increase their populations but to hold their market share under circumstances that are increasingly competitive. Under these circumstances, some secondary measures of market performance may be appropriate. Some of these might be the extent to which other participants are discouraged from entering into a given market area because of the existing trade patterns supported by the PPO or—and this could be dubious from the point of view of providers—the degree to which the PPO heightens price competition among existing providers in a community. To the provider, a retail discount is not an incentive. The emphasis is on preserving the bottom line, not necessarily through volume but through a better patient mix.

One clear problem that arises—both at the time of formation of the PPO and over time—is designation of the *preferred* provider. Obviously, not every hospital furnishes the same level of care, with the same level of cost-effectiveness. Measures of cost-effectiveness also vary, given the range and acuity of services. Walter McClure, president of the Center for Policy Studies, has voiced the reservation that insurers, due to lack of solid information on charges per patient diagnosis, will form PPOs "simply by signing up any providers that will offer a discount."[15] He is fearful that the result could be the designation of high-priced providers as "preferred." He cautions that PPOs must be careful, in the expansion of their geographical bases, to enlist "only the most cost-effective providers."[16]

Restricting PPO participation only to the cost-effective may also be a problem for employers and insurers. Many believe that over time, employers will experience employee pressure to increase the range of choices, leading to expansion of the number of "preferred" hospitals or physicians for convenience and other reasons. Such expansion may lead to the inclusion of non-cost-efficient providers within a PPO network. Also, a non-cost effective providers may seek to be included in the network, posing organizational and legal problems.

Potential problems

The issue of noncost-efficiency includes a second potential problem: that of price determination. Negotiated fee schedules—as noted in the chapter on legal development—may come under judicial scrutiny for both antitrust and potential price fixing. Under the PPO option, some providers now offer discounts from regular charges, rather than from some community-based average for the same procedure. A "discount" could, in actuality, represent a charge that is significantly above community averages. The cost-effectiveness of a PPO could, then, be dependent upon an employer's knowledge of provider charges and community norms.

Another potential problem exists in the tension created by the needs of providers to maintain utilization rates. The essential question that must be asked is whether providers will escalate their styles of practice despite the incentives PPOs create for utilization review and cost containment.

In the past, the practice of discounting to both HMOs and Blue Cross has created some hardships for hospitals. Given the current federal reimbursement methodology and the practice of cost-shifting, it is clear that the practice of discounting will exacerbate hospitals' fiscal problems. A survey in 1980 of the financial status of hospitals in large cities offers a modicum of optimism: it found that the hospital industry is in sound condition, earning almost 4 per cent on average as total margin.[17] The best indicator of financial stress was found to be a hospital's volume of care to the poor. But care to the poor is a social issue, not a provider survival strategy.

In practice, the PPO must prove that its economies can be justified and not merely by the practice of discounting. The efficacy of the PPO must be proven, over time and in practice, to come from control of utilization, as well as costs, while impinging neither upon quality of that service nor upon reasonable choice and consumer access to care.

The oldest new generation PPO is less than five years old. The survival and success of the individual PPO must be carefully differentiated from that of PPOs as an industry. The PPO industry is in a period of rapid growth. If its history follows that of the HMO model, then there will be industry-wide consolidation, as concept gives way to the practical realities of organizational survival. Such a shakedown may already be happening in California, with the declared insolvency of at least two contracting third-party administrators.

If failure occurs, it seems likely to occur within four areas:

1. Where legal-regulatory requirements are not met;

2. Where organizational failure occurs through poor administration of management;

3. Where there is failure to meet the cost containment objectives of the insurer-purchases of the PPO plan; and

4. Where there is failure in marketing (from ''product design'' to promotion) for all constituents involved in the PPO (a better mousetrap, however, does not guarantee purchase or use).

The PPO, of course, will ultimately measure its success in ways typical of other economic entities. That is, its ability to grow and survive. Participation levels in a PPO can be tabulated and compared with alternative delivery and financing schemes in a given market. It will be important to measure the effectiveness of the PPO movement in general in attracting patients from existing financing systems. Of equal significance will be data that will identify the source of the individuals joining the PPO, including the nature and size of the sponsoring group. Detailed understanding of the population attracted to PPOs will also be important, including demographic distribution by age and sex. One vital question will be whether there is negative selection in a PPO. These data elements will be of critical importance in understanding the roles that PPOs play and in their evaluation.

Another key question in measuring the successes of these programs relates to the nature of the sponsoring organization. It is clear from initial activities in California that control of the payment dollar is more significant than control of the service capability in accelerating the development and operation of a PPO. Provider organizations, while they have focused their attention on combining their marketing with other like-minded entities, have not been as successful as insurers and other payer groups in organizing operational PPOs. A major factor in this is, of course, provider reluctance to commit all marketing efforts to a third-party organization, even when providers are active sponsors and financiers. A specific contractual offer or an invitation-to-participate offer from a major payer in a community—whether it is a self-insurer group, a union trust fund, a Blue Cross plan, or a major insurer—is a powerful disincentive to provider-sponsored groups.

Payer-sponsored groups tend to be particularly focused on seeking price advantage and discounts and are willing to use their leverage in negotiating favorable agreements with selected providers. Communities of providers, on the other hand, do not necessarily view themselves as a collective, since their markets are less likely to be competitive within a PPO and dependent upon a wide range of payment sources.

It can be argued that provider-sponsored groups may find themselves eliminated in a second round of contracting, once relationships have been established by the individual provider with a specific payor. While this is likely to occur in reference to certain payor groups, it is clear that provider-sponsored groups do offer the advantages of organization and potential for stronger utilization review than would be likely to emerge from the relatively unsophisticated payor.

A key factor in the early survival of any PPO, of course, is the nature of its financing. This has been a critical problem, particularly in reference to provider-based groups. As these groups continue to struggle with the questions of organization, governance, and initial financing, they may find it increasingly less viable than payor alternatives. This will be particularly crucial, so that the evidence of success at the provider level will be a long time coming. This evidential delay can, of course, be attributed to the factors cited relative to the long chain of decisions before a patient shows up and the difficulty in demonstrating a clear increase or shift in patient case load in mature markets. Survival of a PPO under these circumstances may be linked to other sources of revenues than dues or investments from the sponsoring provider. These potential sources of revenues include an organized utilization review program and/or claims processing system. Both of these, however, require investment and may raise questions relative to certain payor organizations. As noted before, an internally for-profit organized utilization review program may come into question as to its objectivity. A claims processing system may conflict directly with the activity of an insurer, particularly where it also serves as a third-party administrator.

Importance of data collecting and reporting

In looking at the PPO's success, and its ability to hold down costs and market aggressively, it is clear that a system for the collection and reporting of data is critical. As in most emerging activities, however, little focus has been placed upon the need to accumulate information for an effective assessment of the programs. Payers and providers will need to work closely together to ensure that data is not lost early on and that progressive refinement and analysis is supported.

We can only note that PPOs, as they exist today, are the product of analysis. The evidentiary base for their development and justification in the marketplace is at best scant. Despite the eagerness of health care providers and certain health care payers to venture into the preferred provider organization waters, there is a good deal of skittishness and caution about this third-wave in the financing and delivery of health care.

The history of HMO development gives rise, however, to a cautious optimism. If this pattern of development applies to the PPO, a period of rapid growth will be followed by a period of consolidation, where problems are resolved. This will be followed by a period of mature growth and success. The HMO has reached that stage. According to the federal Health and Human Services' Office of Health Maintenance Organizations, a study conducted by Touche Ross and Company found that some 90 per cent of the nation's 60 largest HMOs showed a profit, with returns on equity running as high as 50 per cent. Four years ago, half of the HMOs surveyed were not profitable.

HMOs are now a $6.1 billion industry. Enrollment growth has been more than 11 per cent per year since 1971. The prospects for the PPO as industry are as encouraging as well; the fate of each individual organization rests—as with other business concerns—on the legal, financial and marketing foresight of its developers and the strength of its practical application to local conditions.

The PPO remains relatively untested. If a final determination of its value remains to be made, it is only because it lacks a proven history, and the environment in which it exists is still in flux. The competitive market place gives rise to further innovation, rapid change.

Notes

1. Hunt, David. Preferred Provider Organizations. *Private Practice.* (14)11:19. November 1982.
2. Denver PPOs Save One-Fifth on Bills. *Health Services Information.* (9)30:3. July 5, 1982.
3. *Op. Cit.,* p. 20.
4. Havighurst, Clark C. and Hackbarth, Glenn M. Private Cost Containment. *New England Journal of Medicine.* (300)23:1303. June 7, 1979.

5. Hunt, p. 19.
6. Rundle, Rhonda L. Little Relief in Sight for Soaring Health Premiums. *Business Insurance*. (17)2:3. January 10, 1983.
7. *Ibid.*, p. 3.
8. *Ibid.*, p. 4.
9. A Confidential Survey of Benefit Managers by Segal Associates. Martin E. Segal Company. August 1982.
10. Inglehart, John K. Health Policy Report. *New England Journal of Medicine*. (308)4:233. January 27, 1983.
11. White, Charles H. and Arstein-Kerslake, Cindy. PPO Activity in California Hospitals. *CHA INSIGHT*. (7)22:3. May 26, 1983.
12. *Ibid.*, p. 2.
13. Preferred Provider Organizations: A New Approach to Health Care Delivery. *Interact*. May-June 1983.
14. Kuntz, Esther Fritz. Hospitals Forming PPOs to Fend Off HMO Rivals. *Modern Healthcare*. (13)2:22. February 1983.
15. Hunt, p. 21.
16. Hunt, p. 18.
17. Hadley, Feder and Mullner, pp. 24–25.

CHAPTER ELEVEN

The Future of the PPO

For preferred provider organizations, the future health system offers many alternatives. Perhaps the best thing about these new health care organizations is that so little is known about them, and the PPO can serve as a vehicle for experimentation. Many forms of sponsorship, payment and provider arrangements are possible. The survivors will be those PPO organizations that meet the Darwinian challenge of the marketplace.

Health care in transition

Today's health system is in a major period of transition. Both society and the economy are shifting from an industrial era with substantial government control to a new economic order based on information. There are ten "megatrends" in this changing environment, according to John Naisbitt, author of the best-seller of that title:

Social/Economic "Megatrends"[1]

#1 Industrial Society	Information Society
#2 Forced Technology	High Tech/High Touch
#3 National Economy	World Economy
#4 Short Term	Long Term
#5 Centralization	Decentralization
#6 Institutional Help	Self-Help
#7 Representative Democracy	Participatory Democracy
#8 Hierarchies	Networking
#9 North	South
#10 Either/Or	Multiple-Option

Key trends for the health industry in this social evolution are the shift from an industrial society to an information society, from a national to global economy, and from a short to long-term orientation in social and business investment. Tomorrow's corporations will be decentralized networks, in contrast with the large-scale centralized bureaucracies of the past.[2] In the marketplace, consumers will have multiple options for everything from cable TV stations and services to exotic fruits and vegetables available without regard to season. In the health care marketplace, consumers will have multiple options with regard to price, service, location and convenience, style of practice, and level of personal responsibility for one's own health.

A number of "megatrends" will be driving forces in shaping the health system of the future:

1. **Corporate Model.** Health has been characterized as a "cottage industry," with many small, independent producers. Tomorrow's health organization will be a large, diversified corporation on the private sector model.

2. **Buyers and Sellers.** There will be buyers in the future health market with real purchasing clout, with large-scale health vendors to meet their needs. In addition to government, which has been the largest health care purchaser, private buyers, including major employers and employer coalitions for joint purchasing, large union Taft-Hartley health funds. Consortiums of insurers and intermediaries, will act as "jobbers" for their client group, purchasing health services on volume-discount basis.

3. **Technopush.** Technology will continue to be a major force in the health industry. There will be significant advances in telecommunications, genetic engineering, diagnostic medical imaging, and artificial intelligence. Technology has contributed an estimated 25 percent of rising health costs in the past. Health care organizations will have to decide how much they will be driven by the "technological imperative" to acquire each new technology which becomes available.

4. **Competition.** For the first time, health organizations will compete for economic survival. Price will be a primary factor in the competitive struggle.[3] Strategies for competition will include advertising, affiliating with a large corporation for advantages of scale, or finding a protected market niche. Health organizations will have to decide to position themselves at the "upscale" end of the market, providing premium services and amenities, or follow the private-sector "discounters" with no-frills services at low-end prices.[4]

5. **Conglomerates.** Large-scale, multinational, multibillion dollar corporations will come to dominate much of the

health industry in the next 20 years.[5] In a difficult economy, the conglomerates will be the only ones with access to capital for growth and development on a global basis.

6. **Cost Management.** The survivors in tomorrow's competitive environment will be those health organizations that can control their costs to compete effectively on price. Health organizations will practice "corporate medicine" in defining cost and quality parameters for the delivery of their services.

7. **Vulnerability.** All health organizations will be at risk. There will be market failure of some health organizations, which cannot compete on price nor find a protected market niche.

8. **Flexibility.** The need for innovation will be at a premium in tomorrow's health care market.[6] As the environment changes, health organizations must become very proficient at adaptation, altering their service and product lines as often as needed to meet changing consumer preferences.

9. **Consumerism.** The consumer revolution in health is just beginning. It is part of the "self-help" movement, a shift away from a reliance on social institutions for the solution of human needs.[7] As consumers take more responsibility for their health, they are taking back control over health care decision-making previously dominated by health professionals. Consumers will be more independent, more self-reliant in seeking information and more self-confident in making decisions about their own health.

10. **Value Drift.** As health organizations become more businesslike, they may inadvertently lose their sense of mission and purpose.[8] Preoccupation with the "bottom line"

in a competitive market may result in a loss of touch with the consumer. Successful organizations must stay close to their consumers and not lose their value core of "caring" for real human needs.

Threats and opportunities

The future is a kaleidoscope of threats and opportunities. The best management strategies for one PPO may lead to failure for another. Each developing PPO must be sensitive to this future environment, aware of both the hazards and the opportunities of the future health care market in its strategic planning and management.

There are a number of possible real dangers for the future of Preferred Provider Organizations:

- *Quick Fix.* The PPO may be seen by some sponsors, payors or entrepreneurs as an expedient solution to today's problems. The lack of long-term vision for the PPO leaves it vulnerable to premature termination if it experiences market shifts and developmental problems that are highly likely in the early years. The PPO must be seen as more than a "band-aid" solution.

- *Limited Incentives.* The new PPO possibly will not stimulate any fundamental change in the attitudes or behavior of either consumers or providers. Consumers may be under no incentive—other than financial—to use the PPO and given no incentive to alter or reduce their use of health services.[9] Providers will, in the beginning, share only limited financial risk in the arrangements: their incentives are to gain a greater market share and, thereby, a better mix of patients and better profitability.

- *PPO Failure.* The failure of some PPOs is likely, due to a variety of business hazards. Hospitals, in the early stages, may not have many of the needed skills in marketing and entrepreneurial management. Some PPOs will be poorly designed, others will experience financial losses. Given that there are no statutory requirements for reserves, some payors and providers could be unpaid creditors of bankrupt PPOs. The recent experience of "Multiple Employer Trusts" in California and Washington demonstrates the financial fragility of some of these new health care arrangements.[10]

● *Health Maintenance.*   There is no incentive for health maintenance in the PPO scheme. Consumers gain no benefits from controlling their health services use, and providers only benefit from expanded service demand. If a long-term goal of payors is to improve the health status of their consumers so they require fewer and less intensive services, the PPO will need modification to provide incentives for such behavior.

● *A Fad?*   Are PPOs only a transitory phenomenon? Certainly some skepticism is in order. So far, the PPO concept is long on promise and short on performance. The first "successful" PPO has still had only very limited market penetration, and generates only 4 per cent of the inpatient service demand for its sponsor hospital.[11] Payors have been reluctant to commit to the PPO concept in significant numbers, to date. Expectations for PPO performance should be kept in perspective.

● *Postpones the Real Issues.* There is some valid criticism of the PPO concept, that it fails to confront some of the most fundamental issues between consumer, provider and payor of health services.[12] Some of these issues will occur in the PPO's early development in confrontations around issues of "cost" versus "quality" between the PPO organization, which must control its costs, and it providers, who seek to provide the highest and best level of care available. Consumers and payors are caught directly in the middle of that controversy. More than one developing PPO will founder on these issues.

- *Quality.*   With the dominant emphasis on limiting costs, so the PPO can make a reasonable rate of return at below-market prices, quality may suffer. Utilization review may be seen primarily as a mechanism to keep service use down, rather than protecting a "floor" of acceptable quality. HMOs have dealt successfully with the quality protection issue but have had more incentive to do so, since HMOs have a long-range and contractual relationship with their consumers. PPOs will have to be sensitive to the quality issue.

- ***Lack of Regulatory Oversight.***   At this early stage, PPOs are not covered by any federal regulation and by state regulation in only a few states (see chapter 9). There are certainly dangers in this lack of regulatory oversight. California's experience with "Prepaid Health Plans" for Title 19 Medi-Cal beneficiaries in the early 1970s indicates that unscrupulous operators will take advantage of unregulated businesses.[13] On the other hand, premature regulation—prior to experience with the problems and the potential of the PPO concept—could have a dampening effect upon this promising new organizational form.

For the future PPO, there will be opportunities to achieve goals of all three parties at interest—providers, consumers and payors:

- *Savings.*   The primary interest of PPO purchasers is the potential for reducing health expenditures. The more their consumers choose the PPO, the greater the savings over more costly fee-for-service care.

- *Control.*   There are two ways PPOs will reduce costs— through discount payments to providers and in the potential they offer for greater control over utilization. Discounts are only effective during the initial phase of competition. If prices settle at a new, lower level, the PPO must then compete on its ability to control both the type and level of service by the consumer. The PPO advantage over traditional insurance plans, as well as over HMOs, is its flexibility. The PPO can design health service plans that are tailored to the budgets and preferences of its major purchasers, and even build the purchaser into the utilization review process.

- *Network.*   The PPO concept can be packaged and marketed through a network of preferred provider organizations, on a statewide, regional and national basis.[14] Not-for-profit and proprietary health care systems have an excellent potential to negotiate large-scale contracts with national employers or with consortia of local or statewide employers. Franchising offers a ready alternative for marketing the PPO on a state, regional or national basis. Sponsorship on a statewide basis by an insuror, Blue Cross, is already being marketed aggressively in California.

- *Flexibility.*   There are practically no rules for the PPO arrangement. Its sponsorship, pricing, administration, provider relations, utilization review, consumer incentives, and other features are not fixed by tradition or regulation.

- *Customized Benefits.*   Each PPO may be unique to its environment and the interests of the three major parties. In this early stage, we have little background upon which to judge what will or will not work. This may provide the license for PPO designers to break with tradition, eliminating parameters such as "full coverage for inpatient care," or including non-traditional services such as biofeedback. A company with a large number of employees who have experienced back problems, for example, may design a program with its PPO to provide prevention, education and health promotion, and fitness programs directed towards reducing worker's compensation as well as health costs.

- *Competition.* The advent of preferred provider organizations will stimulate competition in the health marketplace in three directions: with traditional sources of health services of insurance; with other PPOs; and with health maintenance organizations (HMO).[15] In an already competitive market, the Twin Cities metropolis in Minnesota, the seven established HMOs are being undercut on price by new PPOs.[16] The PPOs believe they can take business away from the less flexible HMOs, and the HMOs can be expected to counter. Competition is only beginning.

- *Partnerships.* The PPO provides an opportunity to break with tradition in the organization, payment and delivery of health services. As the first innovation in health care financing in a decade, it gives purchasers, providers and payors a clean slate on which to design the health care organization of the future.

Three future scenarios

Of the many possible futures for health, three scenarios for the health system in the year 2000 illustrate the potential of this new organizational arrangement, the preferred provider organization.[17]

The first scenario, *"High Technology,"* extends the progress in treating and preventing disease through advances in biomedical technology. There will be "super drugs" targeted to receptor sites on cells to cure cancer and other diseases without surgery. Not only will organ transplants be commonplace, but micro-mini computers will be implanted to direct their activities. Artificial joints will replace damaged natural parts. Genetic engineering may make it possible for children born after 1990 to live to be 150 years old. Medical technology will be widely available, and the American health system will grow through multi-national corporations delivering health care technology across the world. The "information revolution" will link consumers and providers through low-cost two-way communications.

Under this scenario for the health system of the future, we can imagine a scenario for PPOs entitled *"Upscale PPO."* This PPO is designed to appeal to the "upscale" consumer—affluent, well-educated and discriminating. The PPO would provide a broadly comprehensive package of services, such as personalized follow-up after services to check post-treatment satisfaction. The PPO package would include special health promotion and fitness services, through a network of health/fitness spas. Two-way communications would provide education and advice/ consultation to consumers from the PPO provider network to consumers in their homes or offices. In this package, the full array of high technology medicine would be applied, with minimum concern for cost considerations except for procedures considered cosmetic. Employers would purchase the "Upscale PPO" package as a desirable form of executive compensation. The "Upscale PPO" would be available internationally, for an elite clientele who can afford and seek the very best that technology and the health system has to offer.

In the second scenario, *"Conglomerates,"* a fundamental restructuring of the health industry occurs. In a process of acquisition and corporate growth that parallels development of multinational firms in the private sector in the 1960s, the health industry comes to be dominated by a handful of very large companies. By the year 2000, more than 90 per cent of all hospitals are members of multi-institutional systems. Several of the largest for-profit systems have themselves become part of larger conglomerates, being acquired by companies like General Foods.

The PPO scenario driven by the vision of future "conglomerates" is the *"PPO Network."* The new conglomerates are both horizontally and vertically integrated systems of local and regional PPOs. PPOs are the building blocks of the health conglomerate. Each PPO is unique, providing a complete package of services to enrollees and corporations in its market. Prepayment on a capitation basis is the dominant mode of financing. Some employers and insurance companies still prefer to pay on a fee-for-service basis, a mode which is rapidly disappearing. PPOs compete, sometimes intra-company, with different levels of service packages from basic "no-frills" to deluxe.

The third scenario, *"Wellness,"* assumes a basic transformation in consumer attitudes and health behavior. The lifestyle known as "Voluntary Simplicity" becomes a majority consensus. Consumers take more responsibility for their own health. The health promotion providers, who had been on the fringe of the health marketplace, become mainstream providers. Inpatient days fall below 300 per thousand population, and physician visits drop to less than 3 per year. Virtually no one dies in the hospital. Most of the elderly die at home or in hospices.

The *"Live-Well" PPO* embodies the new paradigm of health which drives the "Wellness" scenario of the future. This PPO network is strongly decentralized. At its base are the alternative healers and therapists who provide holistic and human-centered services to PPO consumers. Organized as an alternative to hospital-based PPOs, the "Live-Well" program has caught the imagination of consumers dissatisified with bureaucratic medicine. Despite it casual organizational structure, the Live-Well program is a financial success because it makes relatively little use of higher cost resources, such as inpatient care. Employers like the program. Employee morale is up and costs are down. "Live-Well" is a flourishing PPO alternative.

The future of PPOs according to the experts

Which of these scenarios will be successful? In their extreme, none will become *the* future. Elements of each will contribute to a future for health care, a new synthesis of current trends.

The future of the PPO concept may be bright, but it is not yet clear. In Greek mythology, when the gods had a difficult question about the future, they sought the advice of the Oracle at Delphi. In modern futures research, the ''Delphi'' poll asks a panel of experts to provide their best estimates of the future. The intersection of the opinions of a diverse set of experts may illuminate the possible futures of the preferred provider organization.

Dr. Paul Ellwood (Interstudy, Minneapolis)
The most successful hospitals and medical staffs will be participating in at least one PPO within the next three or four years.[18] Any new venture of this type ought to distribute power and ownership in a manner that matches the economic risks for the providers involved. Whatever the arrangement, it must be dynamic and capable of changing as the payment systems change. This new organization must be capable of coping with the individual payor's unique approach to payment. The scheme we've conceived is called ''MESH''—Medical Staff Hospital Development Corporation (See Appendix A). The central MESH organization creates a series of subcorporations, each of which relate directly to individual payors and the set of providers which will service them. Each plan is semi-autonomous and highly flexible. The time is short for hospitals to enter into these new arrangements with their medical staffs—no more than 18 months from the present.

Robert Finney (Hewlett-Packard, Palo Alto, California)
The PPO provides an opportunity for cooperation between doctors, hospitals and businesses to develop cost-effective arrangements that offer quality health care.[19] Businesses want to do more than just respond to proposals. They want to have an impact on PPO development, as a stakeholder rather than just a purchaser. This can be more readily accomplished when the PPO is new and/or small, so the employer can really customize

its plan to meet its needs. PPOs will provide a mini-laboratory for an employer to introduce changes in its benefits program. Successful innovations can be transferred to the corporations' health benefits structure, in other corporate sites or company-wide. Hewlett-Packard has a data base of its health experience upon which to base PPO reimbursement. This will be a quantum leap past negotiation of discounts on fee-schedules. The benefits to businesses—savings aside—will be an enhanced understanding of how the health system functions upon which to develop more effective cost management approaches.

Dr. Steve Moore, former medical director for SAFECO, Seattle, Washington
The PPO movement can benefit from the experiences of both successful and failed HMOs.[20] One of the greatest dangers for a health care organization coming into a community is to try to impose a system—especially a new system—without an understanding of the local environment. PPOs must be designed consistent with the traditions and needs of the community. Both providers and purchasers should recognize that the PPO is no panacea and cannot achieve short-term miracles.

Peter Fox—Lewin Associates, Washington, D.C.
In the life cycle of a PPO, the organization starts with few financial problems.[21] Then it experiences rising costs. The response is to tighten controls and revise financial arrangements. The outcome will either be effective organizational control over providers, or PPO failure. In the future, a PPO's efficiency will come through control of services, not just as a product of discounting provider reimbursement.

PPOs will need solid data to justify their efficiency claim, to be successful in marketing the PPO concept. Collaboration will promote PPO success, by sharing financial risks with providers and through involvement of purchasers in provider selection.

William A. Guy, Office of the Governor, Sacramento, California
Selective provider purchasing is the most dramatic change in the health care system since the invention of health insurance—changes which may not make doctors or hospitals very happy.[22] The State of California's experimental Selective Provider Contracting Program is an alternative to public utility regulation of the health industry. If the State of California can save $100 million per year through the PPO approach, this will lead California toward a long-term commitment to a competitive approach for reducing health costs. This program does not guarantee the solvency of hospitals. That was the old system. But prospective payment will help hospitals and physicians in the long run.

Robert Burnett, M.D.—LIFEGUARD, Santa Clara, California
Physicians must take the lead in PPO development.[23] The alternative is to allow an insurance company or a large corporation to control medicine—to tell doctors how to practice medicine. If they refuse, the payor will not contract with them. Fee-for-service medicine is not dead, but the trend will be toward contractual relationships between purchaser and provider. The medical community can respond by organizing itself as a corporate entity, and taking the initiative with the major employers and insurors.

Lawrence W. Margolis—Herman Smith Associates, Hinsdale, Illinois
With the burgeoning interest in PPOs, we can expect more competition across the health industry.[24] Insurers will form preferred provider organizations and exclusive provider organizations if hospitals and physicians do not move quickly to gain the initiative. If insurers form PPOs and EPOs, hospital's revenues will drop more quickly than if the facilities are the PPO sponsors or managers. Even if a PPO increases a hospital's business by only a few percentage points, the relationship will help the hospital

keep its current volume in an increasingly competitive market. The demand for hospital services will be altered by PPOs, and physicians' attitudes will change. They will become more competitive with non-participating institutions and each other, and they may become more willing to work for other alternative delivery systems, such as Health Maintenance Organizations.

Conclusion

While the future is never perfectly clear, a number of key trends are already evident which will have a powerful effect on tomorrow's health care system. The preferred provider organization is a vehicle for change. It is a transitional mechanism, towards new forms of health organizations, new styles of medical practice, new patterns of health expenditures, and perhaps even a new definition of the business of "health" care delivery.

There has not been such excitement in the health industry since the passage of Medicare and Medicaid, nearly 20 years ago. PPOs have galvanized the industry. Competitive forces are being unleashed, and creative energies are flowing. A new generation of health care organizations is coming—the preferred provider organizations.

Two words of advice:

Get ready.

Notes

1. Naisbitt, John. *Megatrends*. New York: Warner Books. 1982.
2. Office of Technology Assessment, Medical Technology Under Proposals to Increase Competition in Healthcare. U.S. Government Printing Office. Washington, D.C. 1982.
3. Stockman, David A. Premises for a Medical Marketplace: A Neo Conservative's Vision of How to Transform the Health System. *Health Affairs*. Winter 1981.
4. Koehn, Hank. Networking. Lutheran Hospital System Conference on Networking. Phoenix, Arizona. February 20, 1983.

5. Johnson, Richard L. Health Care 2000 A.D.: The Impact of Conglomerates. *Hospital Progress*. April 1981.
6. Kaiser, Leland R. Innovation in the Hospital. *Hospital Forum*. March-April, 1982; Dennis Strum, *et al,* An R&D System that Works: Lutheran Hospital Society Shares its Step-By-Step Process in Building its High-Results Program. *Hospital Forum*. March-April 1982.
7. Anderson, A. R. Nonprofits: Check Your Attention to Customers. *Harvard Business Review*. May-June 1982.
8. Cunningham, Robert M., Jr. Changing Philosophies in Medical Care and the Rule of the Investor-Owned Hospital. *New England Journal of Medicine*. September 23, 1982.
9. Kopp, Walter C. Selective Contracting: Preparing Hospitals and Physicians. Arthur Young and Co. San Francisco. 1983.
10. Keppel, Bruce. Multiple-Employer Trusts Cause Concern: New Insurance Chief Vows to Monitor Health Plans. *LA Times*. May 3, 1983.
11. Johnson, Donald E. L. If Hospitals and Physicians Don't Grab the PPO Market, Insurers Will. *Modern Healthcare*. March 1983.
12. Berger, Judith D. Selective Contracting: California's Hot Potato? *Hospital Forum*. November-December 1982.
13. Maloney, Sheila A. Preferred Provider Organizations: An Overview for State Regulations. *The New Times*. National Association of Health Maintenance Organization Regulators. March 1, 1983.
14. Johnson, Donald E. L. Nonprofit Networks Link Resources to Grab Piece of National Markets. *Modern Healthcare*. October 1982.
15. O'Connor, Maureen L. Preferred Provider Organizations: A Market Approach to Healthcare Competition. *Hospital Forum*. November-December 1982.
16. Kuntz, Esther Fritz. Hospitals Forming PPOs to Fend off HMO Rivals. *Modern Healthcare*. February 1983.
17. Tibbitts, Samuel J. Healthcare Heads for Revolutionary Changes in Organization, Delivery. *Modern Healthcare*. July 1983.
18. Ellwood, Paul M., M.D. New Organizational Arrangements to Help Doctors and Hospitals Code with HMOs, PPOs, DRGs and Medi-Cal. Presentation to Alternative Healthcare, Delivery Sys-

tems and Medicare in the 1980's. Universal City, California. January 27, 1983.

19. Finney, Robert. Interview. August 9, 1983.
20. Moore, Steve, M.D. Containing Healthcare Costs Through Alternative Delivery Systems: The PPO Approach. Seminar of Healthcare Purchasors of Puget Sound. April 20, 1983.
21. Fox, Peter. Preferred Provider Organizations: A Progress Report. Associated Hospital Systems Trustee, Educational Conference on Private Sector Initiatives to Control Health Costs. Carefree, Arizona. March 15, 1983.
22. Johnson, Donald E. L. Price Competition Will be Legacy of California's Medi-Cal Czar. *Modern Healthcare*. September 1982.
23. Cassidy, Robert. Will the PPO Movement Freeze You Out? *Medical Economics*. April 18, 1983.
24. Johnson, Donald E. L. If Hospitals and Physicians Don't Grab the PPO Market, Insurers Will. *Modern Healthcare*. March 1983.

APPENDIX A
Organizational Prototypes

"Super Messenger" Approach

Exhibit A.1 outlines the "Super Messenger" approach to PPOs. In this arrangement, the PPO represents hospitals and physicians, serving as the providers' marketing agent. Antitrust law prohibits PPO price negotiation on behalf of its providers. Individual providers negotiate directly with payors, or the PPO transmits an offer to the providers, who decide whether or not to buy into the offer. Claims are paid directly to providers by the third-party administrator (TPA). Universal Health Network is an example of this approach.

Particularly in the case of physicians, individual contracting has the limitation of creating a burdensome system by which each physician must agree to a payor's offer. One method of minimizing this problem may be a services agreement provision to allow automatic acceptance of the offer within a specific time period.

It is also important that PPO acceptance of the payor's offer hinge upon the achievement of a certain level of participation (e.g., 60 per cent) of PPO members.

A major advantage of the "Super Messenger" approach is that it is relatively uncomplicated and inexpensive to implement.

Exhibit A.1
"Super Messenger" Approach

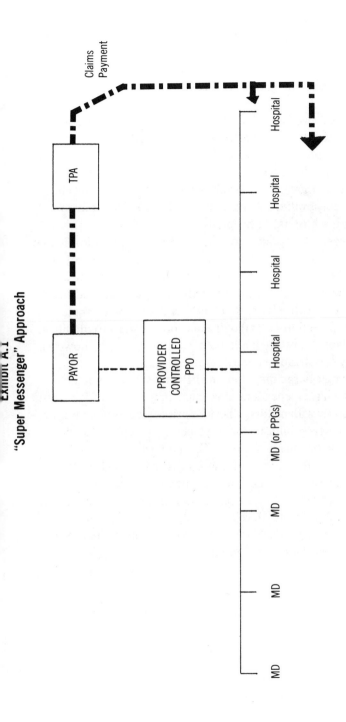

Claims Payment

TPA

PAYOR

PROVIDER CONTROLLED PPO

MD   MD   MD   MD (or PPGs)   Hospital   Hospital   Hospital   Hospital

Fully or Partially Integrated Approach

Exhibit A.2 profiles the second major PPO configuration in which physicians are organized in professional practice groups (PPGs).

Organizational options for the PPG include an unincorporated association, partnership, for-profit corporation, tax-exempt entity, or taxable corporation. Another approach is an economic joint venture with a hospital or hospitals.

An increasingly attractive option for PPG organization is the professional corporation (PC), which provides more certainty regarding some legal issues and more liability protection since only assets of the corporation, not the individual, are affected in the event of loss. One disadvantage of a PC is that all of its employees are subject to Section 414(m) of the tax code, requiring equality in pension plans. This need not be a stumbling block, however, particularly for already established group practices.

To be a single bargaining unit, the PPO must be as integrated as possible. If it has independent economic significance, the PPO can bargain directly with payors, otherwise price-fixing problems arise. The third party-administrator pays claims to the PPO, which distributes the payments to the PPGs and hospitals.

The obvious advantage of this approach is the PPO's ability to negotiate on behalf of physicians, who are organized in the PPGs. Physicians not already participating in a group practice may be somewhat reluctant to develop PPGs, constituting the major drawback of this approach. PPGs can, incidentally, be incorporated in the "Super Messenger" model.

Exhibit A.2
Fully or Partially Integrated Approach

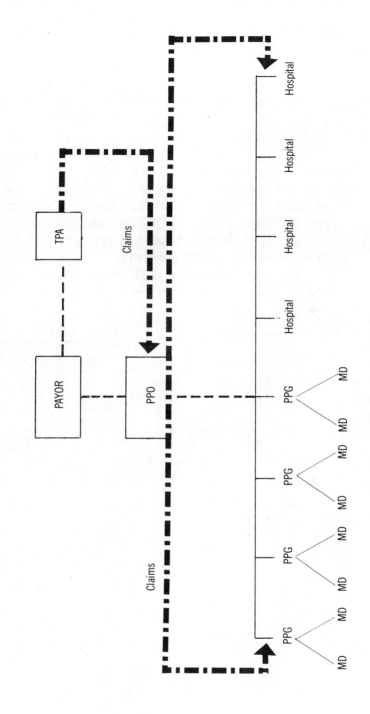

Hospital(s)-Based PPO with Minority Physician Participation

Yet another organizational option, described in exhibit A.3, is the formation of a new PPO entity, such as a corporation, which is controlled by the hospital.

Physicians are represented by this entity. In this model, the PPO negotiates price terms with individual physicians and then negotiates with payor on behalf of the physician network with each hospital. Claims are paid directly to hospitals by the TPA, while the PPO receives payments that are then distributed to participating physicians. Understandably, the major determinant of the feasibility of this option is the degree to which physicians choose to be active participants in the PPO.

Exhibit A.3
Hospital Controlled PPO with
Minority Physician Participation

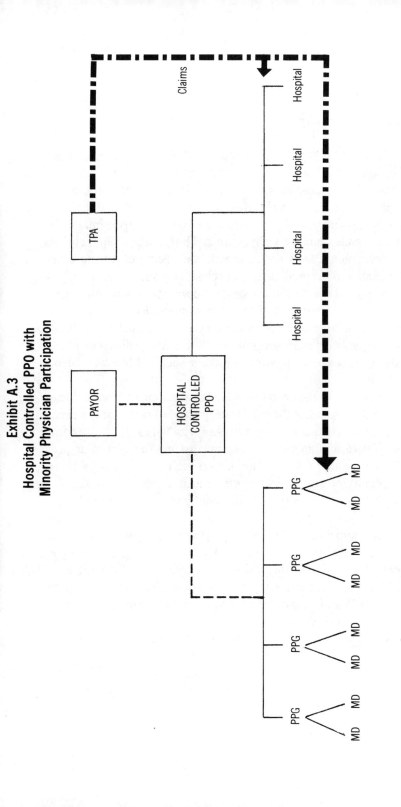

"MESH" Approach

Proposed by Paul M. Ellwood, Jr., director of the prestigious Minnesota thinktank, InterStudy, MESH is an acronym for a Medical Staff Hospital joint venture development corporation. Conceptually, MESH seeks to link common interests and concerns of hospitals and their medical staffs in flexible arrangements, based on the premise that every physician and hospital participant in any payment plan affects the economic well being of all the other physician and hospital participants in that plan.

Through the joint venture or development corporation, hospitals and their medical staff jointly and equitably participate in a variety of price-sensitive payment arrangements, such as a PPO. A series of subcorporations, potentially involving different physicians, can thus relate to various payors, such as Medicare, Medicaid, etc.

Integration of the hospital and medical staff in this manner may raise issues relating to the corporate practice of medicine and needs to be evaluated against state laws. Antitrust issues might also come into play, although these arrangements may be viewed as pro-competitive and in the economic and health care interests of the community, critical mitigating elements in antitrust analysis.

Exhibit A.4 shows the possible configuration of a MESH preferred provider organization. To date, this innovative concept has not been implemented for PPOs; however, its flexible, cooperative, and logical approach warrants close investigation. The involvement of the hospital medical staff is tantamount for MESH to succeed. Physician eligibility criteria would need to be centralized in the PPO and hospital medical staff bylaws would have to be supportive of these criteria.

Exhibit A.4
"MESH" Approach

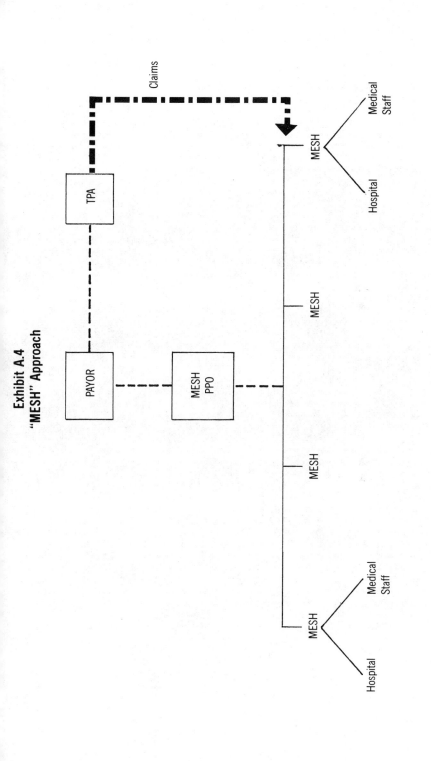

APPENDIX B

Blue Cross of California Participating Hospital Agreement*

*The material in this section related to sample contracts appears with the cooperation and permission of the Blue Cross of California. We thank that organization for its help in making this available.

BLUE CROSS OF CALIFORNIA

PARTICIPATING HOSPITAL AGREEMENT

TABLE OF CONTENTS

EXHIBITS

BLUE CROSS OF CALIFORNIA

PARTICIPATING HOSPITAL AGREEMENT

This AGREEMENT is effective on _____, 1983, between BLUE CROSS OF
CALIFORNIA ("BLUE CROSS") and _____ ("HOSPITAL").

I.   RECITALS

1.1   BLUE CROSS is a California non-profit hospital service corporation,
       duly licensed by the Insurance Commissioner of the State of California,
       pursuant to Insurance Code Section 11495 et seq., to issue benefit
       agreements covering the provision of health care services and to enter
       into agreements with HOSPITAL.

1.2   HOSPITAL is a California corporation, qualified under California
       Insurance Code Sections 11501 and 11502, and duly licensed by the State
       Department of Health Services to provide general acute inpatient and
       outpatient hospital services for Blue Cross Members.

1.3   HOSPITAL provides health care services that meet all legal standards
       of care. HOSPITAL meets the standards of the Joint Commission on
       Accreditation of Hospitals, is certified to participate in the Medicare
       program under Title XVIII of the Social Security Act, and complies with
       with all applicable Federal, State and local laws.

1.4   BLUE CROSS intends by entering into this Agreement to make available
       quality health care to Blue Cross Prudent Buyer Members by contracting
       with HOSPITAL. HOSPITAL intends to provide such quality health care in
       a cost-efficient manner.

II. DEFINITIONS

2.1   "Benefit Agreement(s)" means the written agreement entered into by BLUE
       CROSS and groups or individuals under which BLUE CROSS provides,
       indemnifies, or administers health care benefits.

2.2   "Day of Service" means a measure of time during which a Member receives
       hospital services and which occurs when a Member occupies an inpatient
       acute care bed as of 12:00 midnight or when a Member is admitted and
       discharged within the same day, provided that such admission and
       discharge are not within twenty-four (24) hours of a prior discharge.

2.3   "Emergency" means a sudden onset of a medical condition manifesting itself by acute symptoms of sufficient severity that the absence of immediate medical attention could reasonably result in:

    (1)   permanently placing the Member's health in jeopardy,

    (2)   causing other serious medical consequences,

    (3)   causing serious impairment to bodily functions, or

    (4)   causing serious and permanent dysfunction of any bodily organ or part.

2.4   "Hospital Services" means those acute care inpatient and hospital outpatient services which are covered by a Prudent Buyer Benefit Agreement. Hospital Services do not include long term non-acute care.

2.5   "Medically Necessary" means services or supplies which, under the provisions of this Agreement, are determined to be:

    (1)   Appropriate and necessary for the symptoms, diagnosis or treatment of the medical condition, and

    (2)   Provided for the diagnosis or direct care and treatment of the medical condition, and

    (3)   Within standards of good medical practice within the organized medical community, and

    (4)   Not primarily for the convenience of the Member, the Member's physician or another provider, and

    (5)   The most appropriate supply or level of service which can safely be provided. For hospital stays, this means that acute care as an inpatient is necessary due to the kind of services the Member is receiving or the severity of the Member's condition, and that safe and adequate care cannot be received as an outpatient or in a less intensified medical setting.

2.6   "Medical Services" means those services provided by a Participating Physician and covered by a Prudent Buyer Benefit Agreement.

2.7   "Member(s)" means Subscribers or enrolled dependents covered by a Prudent Buyer Benefit Agreement.

2.8   "Prudent Buyer Benefit Agreement" means a Benefit Agreement pursuant to which Members have a financial incentive to use Participating Providers.

2.9   "Participating Hospital" means a hospital which has entered into an agreement to provide Hospital Services as a Participating Provider.

2.10 "Participating Physician" means a physician who has entered into an agreement to provide Medical Services as a Participating Provider and who is a "licensee" as that term is defined in Business and Professions Code Section 2041.

2.11 "Participating Provider" means a hospital, other health facility, physician or other health professional which has entered into an agreement with BLUE CROSS to provide health care services for prospectively determined rates.

2.12 "Subscribers" means individuals who have qualified for and are covered by the provisions of a Prudent Buyer Benefit Agreement.

2.13 "Utilization Review" means a function performed by an organization or entity acting as an agent of BLUE CROSS, and selected by BLUE CROSS to review and approve whether inpatient Hospital Services provided, or to be provided, are Medically Necessary.

2.14 "Per diem" means a measure of payment for a Day of Service.

III. RELATIONSHIP BETWEEN BLUE CROSS AND HOSPITAL

3.1   BLUE CROSS and HOSPITAL are independent entities. Nothing in this Agreement shall be construed or be deemed to create a relationship of employer and employee or principal and agent or any relationship other than that of independent parties contracting with each other solely for the purpose of carrying out the provisions of this Agreement.

3.2   Nothing in this Agreement is intended to be construed, or be deemed to create, any right or remedies in any third party, including but not limited to a Member or a Participating Provider other than HOSPITAL.

IV. HOSPITAL SERVICES AND RESPONSIBILITIES

4.1   HOSPITAL shall provide to Members Hospital Services which are Medically Necessary when such services are ordered by a licensed physician or

- 3 -

other licensed health professional and are in accordance with the
applicable Prudent Buyer Benefit Agreement and this Agreement. All
services provided by HOSPITAL to its patients are available to Members.
Such services are listed on Exhibit A, attached to and made part of
this Agreement.

4.2   HOSPITAL shall provide Hospital Services to Members in the same manner
       and quality as those services are provided to all other patients of
       HOSPITAL. Such services shall be provided at locations, the addresses
       of which are listed on Exhibit B, attached to and made part of this
       Agreement. Members shall be accommodated in semi-private rooms unless
       other accommodations are Medically Necessary. If a semi-private room
       is not available then any appropriate accommodations may be used.

4.3   HOSPITAL has, and shall maintain in good standing, all licenses
       required by law, the Certificate of Approval required under Insurance
       Code Section 11501 and 11502, certification to participate in the
       Medicare program under Title XVIII of the Social Security Act, and
       shall maintain the standards of the Joint Commission on Accreditation
       of Hospitals (JCAH). Evidence of maintaining such licenses,
       certificate and standards shall be submitted to BLUE CROSS upon
       request.

4.4   HOSPITAL agrees to participate in the Utilization Review provided in
       Article VII and to abide by decisions resulting from that review
       subject to rights of reconsideration, review and arbitration provided
       in Section 7.5.

4.5   HOSPITAL shall, to the extent possible, seek, accept and maintain
       evidence of assignment for the payment of Hospital Services provided to
       Members by HOSPITAL, under the applicable Prudent Buyer Benefit
       Agreement.

4.6   HOSPITAL shall make a reasonable effort to notify BLUE CROSS within
       five (5) days, whenever the average occupancy of HOSPITAL, based on
       available beds, exceeds ninety (90) percent for any thirty (30) day
       period.

4.7   HOSPITAL shall promptly notify BLUE CROSS of:

       (1) Any changes in its ownership or business address;

       (2) Any legal or governmental action initiated against
            HOSPITAL, including but not limited to an action: (a) for
            professional negligence; (b) for a violation of law; or

- 4 -

(c) against any license, accreditation by JCAH or any successor, or Certificate of Approval required under California Insurance Code Section 11501; which, if successful, would materially impair the ability of HOSPITAL to carry out the duties and obligations of the Agreement.

(3) Any other problem or situation that will materially impair the ability of HOSPITAL to carry out the duties and obligations of this Agreement.

V. BLUE CROSS SERVICES AND RESPONSIBILITIES

5.1 BLUE CROSS agrees to pay HOSPITAL compensation pursuant to the provisions of Article VI.

5.2 BLUE CROSS agrees to grant HOSPITAL the status of "Participating Hospital", to identify HOSPITAL as a Participating Hospital on informational materials to Members, and to direct such Members to HOSPITAL.

5.3 BLUE CROSS agrees to continue listing HOSPITAL as a Participating Hospital until this Agreement terminates pursuant to this Agreement.

5.4 BLUE CROSS agrees to provide HOSPITAL with a list of all Participating Physicians, Participating Hospitals and other Participating Providers.

5.5 BLUE CROSS agrees to provide appropriate identification cards for Members.

VI. COMPENSATION AND BILLING

6.1 HOSPITAL shall seek payment only from BLUE CROSS for the provision of Hospital Services except as provided in Section 6.2. The payment from BLUE CROSS shall be limited to the Per Diem amounts referred to in Section 6.8, less copayments and deductible amounts as provided in Section 6.5.

6.2 HOSPITAL may also seek payment for the provision of Hospital Services from other sources as provided in Section 6.3, and as available pursuant to the coordination of benefit provisions of the applicable Prudent Buyer Benefit Agreement and Section 6.4. In such cases, HOSPITAL may seek payment on a basis other than the rates referred to in Section 6.8.

6.3   HOSPITAL agrees that the only charges for which a Member may be liable
       and be billed by HOSPITAL shall be for Hospital Services not covered
       by the applicable Prudent Buyer Benefit Agreement, for copayments and
       deductible amounts required by the applicable Prudent Buyer Benefit
       Agreement, and as provided in Section 6.10.

6.4   In a case in which BLUE CROSS, under the applicable Prudent Buyer
       Benefit Agreement, is primary under applicable coordination of benefit
       rules provided in Title 10 of the California Administrative Code
       Sections 2232.50 through 2232.56, BLUE CROSS shall pay the Per Diem
       amounts due under this Agreement reduced as provided in Section 6.5.
       In a case in which BLUE CROSS, under the applicable Prudent Buyer
       Benefit Agreement, is other than primary under the coordination of
       benefit rules referred to above, BLUE CROSS shall pay only those
       amounts which when added to amounts received by HOSPITAL from other
       sources, pursuant to the applicable coordination of benefit rules,
       equals one hundred percent of the Per Diem amount required by this
       Agreement.

6.5   BLUE CROSS shall deduct any copayments and deductible amounts required
       by the applicable Prudent Buyer Benefit Agreement from payment due
       HOSPITAL from BLUE CROSS pursuant to this Agreement. Deductions for
       the copayment and deductible amounts shall be determined on the basis
       of HOSPITAL'S itemized billed charges to BLUE CROSS.

6.6   HOSPITAL shall bill BLUE CROSS on forms and in a manner acceptable
       to BLUE CROSS. HOSPITAL shall furnish, on request, all information
       reasonably required by BLUE CROSS to verify and substantiate the
       the provision of Hospital Services and the charges for such services.
       BLUE CROSS reserves the right to review all statements submitted by
       HOSPITAL when necessary.

6.7   BLUE CROSS shall pay HOSPITAL within thirty (30) days of receipt of
       statements which are accurate, complete and otherwise in accordance
       with Section 6.6.

6.8   HOSPITAL shall accept the inpatient Per Diem rate and outpatient
       payment rate set forth in Exhibit C, attached to and made part of this
       Agreement, for inpatient admissions and outpatient visits respectively
       for Hospital Services provided to Members as of the effective date of
       this Agreement. Those rates shall not include payment for those
       physician services listed on Exhibit D attached to and made part of
       this Agreement. HOSPITAL outpatient services provided within twelve
       (12) hours of an inpatient admission and which are related to the
       condition for which the Member is admitted shall be included in the
       inpatient Per Diem rate.

- 6 -

6.9   In the case of an obstetrical admission, HOSPITAL shall count only
       one Day of Service for Hospital Services provided to a Member and her
       newborn. However, in the event that the newborn was in intensive care
       or remained at HOSPITAL beyond the date of the Member's discharge,
       HOSPITAL shall count an additional Day of Service for each Day of
       Service that the newborn was at HOSPITAL or in intensive care.

6.10   HOSPITAL shall not charge Members for Hospital Services denied as not
       being Medically Necessary under Section 7.2, unless HOSPITAL has
       obtained a written waiver from that Member on a form approved by BLUE
       CROSS. Such a waiver shall be obtained in advance of the provision
       of those Hospital Services. The waiver shall clearly state that the
       Member shall be responsible for payment of Hospital Services denied
       by BLUE CROSS.

VII. UTILIZATION REVIEW

7.1   BLUE CROSS shall establish a Utilization Review program which shall
       seek to assure that Hospital Services and Medical Services provided to
       Members are Medically Necessary in an inpatient setting. Utilization
       Review shall follow the procedures provided in Exhibit E, attached to
       and made part of this agreement.

7.2   Utilization Review for inpatient Hospital Services shall include:

       (1)   "Pre-admission review" to determine whether a
             scheduled inpatient admission is Medically
             Necessary. Pre-admission review procedures are
             provided in Exhibit F, attached to and made part
             of this Agreement.

       (2)   "Admission review" to determine whether an
             unscheduled inpatient admission or an admission
             not subject to pre-admission review was Medically
             Necessary.

       (3)   "Concurrent review" to determine whether a
             continued inpatient hospital stay is Medically
             Necessary.

7.3   BLUE CROSS shall conduct retrospective review to determine whether
       outpatient services were Medically Necessary. Any appeal of a decision
       under this section shall be commenced by requesting a review by BLUE
       CROSS. If not satisfied, HOSPITAL may request arbitration as provided
       in Exhibit G, attached to and made part of this Agreement.

7.4   BLUE CROSS shall not retrospectively deny any inpatient services
       approved under Section 7.2.

- 7 -

7.5   HOSPITAL may appeal a Utilization Review decision. The appeal shall
       be commenced by requesting reconsideration by the organization or
       entity making the initial decision. If HOSPITAL is not satisfied with
       that result, it may request a review by BLUE CROSS. If HOSPITAL
       continues not to be satisfied, it may request arbitration as provided
       in Exhibit G.

7.6   HOSPITAL agrees to pay for the cost of Utilization Review within thirty
       (30) days of the date of the billing for such Utilization Review.
       Such cost shall be no greater than thirty dollars ($30) per inpatient
       admission.

7.7   BLUE CROSS agrees to pay for the cost of pre-admission Utilization
       Review when such review determines that an inpatient admission is not
       Medically Necessary.

VIII. RECORDS MAINTENANCE, AVAILABILITY, INSPECTION AND AUDIT

8.1   HOSPITAL shall prepare and maintain all appropriate records on Members
       receiving Hospital Services at HOSPITAL. The records shall be
       maintained in accordance with prudent record-keeping procedures and
       as required by law.

8.2   HOSPITAL agrees to allow review and duplication of any data and other
       records maintained on Members which relate to this Agreement, including
       but not limited to medical records or other records relating to
       billing, payment and assignment. Such review and duplication shall be
       allowed upon reasonable notice during regular business hours and shall
       be subject to all applicable laws and regulations concerning the
       confidentiality of such data or records.

8.3   BLUE CROSS and HOSPITAL agree to keep confidential, and to take all
       reasonable precautions to prevent the unauthorized disclosure of any
       and all records required to be prepared and/or maintained by this
       Agreement.

8.4   Subject to all applicable laws relating to privacy and confidentiality
       requirements, medical records of Members shall be made available upon
       reasonable request to each health professional treating the Member, for
       Utilization Review purposes and to BLUE CROSS.

8.5   Ownership and access to records of Members shall be controlled by
       applicable laws.

IX. LIABILITY,INDEMNITY AND INSURANCE

9.1   Neither BLUE CROSS nor HOSPITAL nor any of their respective agents or employees shall be liable to third parties for any act or omission of the other party.

9.2   HOSPITAL, at its sole expense, agrees to maintain adequate insurance for professional liability and comprehensive general liability. HOSPITAL shall also maintain other insurance as shall be necessary to insure HOSPITAL and its employees against any event or loss which would impair the abilty of HOSPITAL to carry out the terms of this Agreement. Such other insurance shall cover any event or loss that HOSPITAL would protect itself against in absence of this Agreement. In lieu of any insurance, HOSPITAL shall maintain the ability to respond to any and all damages which would be covered by such insurance.

9.3   Upon request by BLUE CROSS, HOSPITAL shall provide BLUE CROSS with copies of insurance policies or evidence of the ability to respond to any and all damages, as provided in Section 9.2.

X. MARKETING, ADVERTISING AND PUBLICITY

10.1   BLUE CROSS shall use its best efforts to encourage Members to use the services of HOSPITAL.

10.2   BLUE CROSS shall have the right to use the name of HOSPITAL for purposes of informing Members and prospective Members of the identity of Participating Hospitals, and otherwise carrying out the terms of this Agreement. HOSPITAL shall have the right to review and approve such use, provided however that such approval shall not be unreasonably denied.

10.3   Except as provided in Section 10.2, BLUE CROSS and HOSPITAL each reserves the right to and the control of the use of its name, symbols, trademarks or service marks presently existing or later established. In addition, except as provided in Section 10.2, neither BLUE CROSS nor HOSPITAL shall use the other party's name, symbols, trademarks or service marks in advertising or promotional materials or otherwise without the prior written consent of that party and shall cease any such usage immediately upon written notice of the party or upon termination of this Agreement, whichever is sooner.

XI. DISPUTE RESOLUTION

11.1   BLUE CROSS and HOSPITAL agree to meet and confer in good faith to resolve any problems or disputes that may arise under this Agreement.

11.2 In the event that any problem or dispute concerning the terms of this
      Agreement, other than a Utilization Review decision as provided for in
      Article VII, is not satisfactorily resolved, BLUE CROSS and HOSPITAL
      agree to arbitrate such problem or dispute. Such arbitration shall be
      initiated by either party making a written demand for arbitration on
      the other party. Within thirty (30) days of that demand, BLUE CROSS
      and HOSPITAL shall each designate an arbitrator and give written notice
      of such designation to the other. Within thirty (30) days after these
      notices have been given, the two arbitrators selected by this process
      shall select a third neutral arbitrator and give notice of the
      selection to BLUE CROSS and HOSPITAL. The three arbitrators shall hold
      a hearing and decide the matter within sixty (60) days thereafter.

11.3 The arbitration shall be conducted pursuant to the California Code of
      Civil Procedure, Title Nine, Section 1280, et seq., unless otherwise
      mutually agreed. HOSPITAL and BLUE CROSS agree that the arbitration
      results shall be binding on both parties in any subsequent litigation
      or other dispute.

XII. TERM AND TERMINATION

12.1 When executed by both parties, this Agreement shall become effective
      as of the date noted on page 1 and shall continue in effect for one
      year. Thereafter this Agreement shall continue in effect until
      terminated pursuant to this Agreement.

12.2 Either party may terminate this Agreement by giving at least one
      hundred and twenty (120) days written notice prior to the expiration
      of the initial one year term. Thereafter, either party may terminate
      this Agreement with or without cause by giving at least one hundred and
      twenty (120) days prior written notice. Nothing in this Agreement
      shall be construed to limit either party's lawful remedies in the event
      of a material breach of this Agreement.

12.3 If this Agreement is terminated, HOSPITAL shall continue to provide and
      be compensated for Hospital Services under the terms of this Agreement
      to Members who are hospital inpatients on the date of termination until
      those Members are discharged.

12.4 Notwithstanding termination, BLUE CROSS shall continue to have access
      to records for four (4) years from the date of provision of the
      Hospital Services to which the records refer. The records shall be
      available in accordance with Article VIII, to the extent permitted
      by law and as necessary to fulfill the terms of this Agreement.

12.5 After the effective date of termination, this Agreement shall remain
      in effect for the resolution of all matters unresolved as of that
      date.

12.6 Renegotiation of the price terms of this contract may be commenced by either party upon written notice at least thirty (30) days prior to the anniversary date of the contract. If agreement on new price terms has not been reached by the anniversary date of the contract, the current rate shall continue in effect until such time as agreement is reached or the contract is terminated.

XIII. UNFORESEEN CIRCUMSTANCES

13.1 In the event that the operations of HOSPITAL's facilities are substantially interrupted by acts of war, fire, insurrection, riots, earthquakes or other acts of nature or any cause that is not the fault of HOSPITAL or is beyond reasonable control of HOSPITAL, HOSPITAL shall be relieved of its obligations only as to those affected operations and only as to those affected portions of this Agreement for the duration of such interruption.

13.2 In the event that the Hospital Services provided by HOSPITAL are substantially interrupted pursuant to an event described in Section 13.1, BLUE CROSS shall have the right to terminate this Agreement upon thirty (30) days' prior written notice to HOSPITAL. Such termination shall be cancelled if BLUE CROSS in its judgment determines that the Hospital Services can be performed in spite of the event or because the interruption has ended. BLUE CROSS shall not unreasonably refuse to cancel such termination.

XIV. GENERAL PROVISIONS

14.1 Assignment

No assignment of the rights, duties, or obligations of this Agreement shall be made by HOSPITAL without the express written approval of a duly authorized representative of BLUE CROSS. Any attempted assignment in violation of this provision shall be void as to BLUE CROSS.

14.2 Subcontracting

HOSPITAL shall not subcontract this Agreement or any portion of it without the prior written consent of BLUE CROSS if the subcontract requires a Member to occupy an inpatient bed or receive Hospital Services at locations other than those listed in Exhibit B. Such consent shall not be unreasonably withheld.

14.3 Waiver of Breach

Waiver of a breach of any provision of this Agreement shall not be deemed a waiver of any other breach of the same or different provision.

14.4 Notices

Any notice required to be given pursuant to the terms and provisions of this Agreement shall be in writing, postage prepaid, and shall be sent by certified mail, return receipt requested, to BLUE CROSS or HOSPITAL at the address below. The notice shall be effective on the date indicated on the return receipt.

> Provider Contracting Department
> Nineteenth Floor
> Blue Cross of California
> 1950 Franklin Street
> Oakland, California 94659

and to HOSPITAL at:

14.5 Severability

In the event any provision of this Agreement is rendered invalid or unenforceable by any valid Act of Congress or of the California Legislature or by any regulation duly promulgated by officers of the United States or of the State of California acting in accordance with law, or declared null and void by any court of competent jurisdiction, the remainder of the provisions of this Agreement shall, subject to paragraph 14.6, remain in full force and effect.

14.6 Effect of Severable Provision

In the event that a provision of this Agreement is rendered invalid or unenforceable or declared null and void as provided in Section 14.5 and its removal has the effect of materially altering the obligations of either BLUE CROSS or HOSPITAL in such manner as, in the judgment of the party affected, (a) will cause serious financial hardship to such party; or (b) will cause such party to act in violation of its corporate Articles or Bylaws, the party so affected shall have the right to terminate this Agreement upon thirty (30) days' prior written notice to the other party. The provisions of Article XII shall apply to such termination.

14.7 Entire Agreement

This Agreement, together with exhibits, contains the entire Agreement
between BLUE CROSS and HOSPITAL relating to the rights granted and the
obligations assumed by the parties concerning the provision of Hospital
Services to Members. Any prior agreements, promises, negotiations or
representations, either oral or written, relating to the subject matter
of this Agreement not expressly set forth in this Agreement are of no
force or effect.

14.8 Amendment

This Agreement or any part or section of it may be amended at any time
during the term of the Agreement by mutual written consent of duly
authorized representatives of BLUE CROSS and HOSPITAL.

14.9 Attorneys' Fees

In the event that either BLUE CROSS or HOSPITAL institutes any action,
suit, or arbitration proceeding to enforce the provisions of this
Agreement, the prevailing party shall recover costs and reasonable
attorneys' fees.

14.10 Headings

The headings of articles and sections contained in this Agreement are
for reference purposes only and shall not affect in any way the meaning
or interpretation of this Agreement.

14.11 Governing Law

This Agreement shall be construed and enforced in accordance with the
laws of the State of California.

BLUE CROSS OF CALIFORNIA   _____
                                                     (Hospital)

By:_____   By:_____

Title:_____   Title:_____

Date:_____   Date:_____

HOSPITAL SERVICES INVENTORY

Line No.	HOSPITAL SERVICES	(1) Code		(2) Code		(3) Code
	DAILY HOSPITAL SERVICES		ANCILLARY SERVICES		CLINIC SERVICES	
005	Coronary Intensive Care		Delivery Room Services		Cardiology	
010	Pediatric Intensive Care		Labor Room Services		Chest Medical	
015	Burn Intensive Care		Alternate Birth Center		Communicable Disease	
020	Medical Intensive Care		Abortion Services		Dermatology	
025	Surgical Intensive Care		Dental Surgery		Diabetes	
030	Newborn Intensive Care		Podiatry Surgery		Allergy	
035	Isolation Intensive Care		Urologic Surgery		Metabolic	
040	Psychiatric Isolation Intensive Care		Otolaryngologic Surgery		Neurology	
045	Pulmonary Intensive Care		Plastic Surgery		Pediatric	
050	Communicable Disease Isolation Care		Surgical Day Care (One Day)		Neonatal	
055	Protective Isolation Care		Gynecologic Surgery		Psychiatric	
060	Definitive Observation Care		Kidney Transplant Services		Obstetrics	
065	Drug Abuse Care		Open Heart Surgery Services		Hypertension	
070	Alcoholism Care		Heart Cath/Sterile Room Service		Rheumatic	
075	Inpatient Care Under Custody (Jail)		Cystoscopy Service		Renal	
080	Metabolic Care		Neurological Surgery		Orthopedic	
085	Newborn Nursery Care		Ophthalmologic Surgery		Trauma Ortho	
090	Mental Retarded Nursery Care		Orthopedic Surgery		Ophthalmology	
095	Premature Nursery Care		Renal Dialysis Services		Otolaryngology	
100	Stroke Care		Anesthesia Services—Surgical		Podiatry	
105	Neonatal Acute Care		Anesthesia Services—Obstetrics		Dental	
110	Post Partum Care		Anatomic Pathologic Services		Alcoholism	
115	Psychiatric Acute Care		Hematologic Services		Child Diagnosis	
120	Pediatric Acute Care		Clinical Chemistry Services		Child Treatment	
125	Geriatric Acute Care		Serologic Services		Drug Abuse	
130	Medical Acute Care		Urinalysis Services		Family Therapy	
135	Surgical Acute Care		Microbiologic Services		Group Therapy	
140	Skilled Nursing/Extended Care		Necropsy Services		OTHER SERVICES	
145	Psychiatric Long-Term Care		Pulmonary Lab Services		Toxicology/Antidote Info	
150	Tuberculosis Long-Term Care		Organ Bank		Drug Reaction Info	
155	Intermediate Care		Blood Bank		Cancer/Tumor Registry	
160	Rehabilitation Care		Electroencephalography		Family Planning	
165	Residential/Custodial Care		Electrocardiography		Genetic Counseling	
170	Mental Retardation Care		Electromyography		Dietetic Counseling	
175	Self Care		X-ray Examination		Parent Training Class	
180	Hospice		X-ray Therapy		Diabetic Training Class	
185	PARTIAL DAY CARE		Cobalt Therapy		Renal Dialysis Training Class	
190	Psychiatric Night Care		Radium Therapy		Public Health Class	
195	Psychiatric Day Care		Diagnostic Radioisotope		Medical Research	
200	HOME CARE SERVICES		Therapeutic Radioisotope		MEDICAL EDUCATION PROGRAMS	
205	Home Physical Medicine Care		Computerized Axial Tomography		Approved Residency	
210	Home Social Service Care		Full Body		Approved Internship	
215	Home Dialysis Training		Partial		Approved Externship	
220	Jail Care		Pharmacy W/FT Registered Pharmacist		Physician's Assistant	
225	Psychiatric Foster Home Care		Pharmacy W/PT Registered Pharmacist		RN	
230	Home Nursing Care		Clinical Pharmacologic Services		LVN	
235	EMERGENCY SERVICES		Psychopharmacological Therapy		Nurse Anesthetist	
240	Emergency Room Service		Shock Therapy		Medical Technologist	
245	Ambulance Service		Physical Therapy		Inhalation Therapist	
250	Mobile Cardiac Care Service		Occupational Therapy		Occupational Therapist	
255	Psychiatric Emergency Service		Speech Therapy		Pharmacy Intern	
260	Emergency Observation Service		Rehabilitation Therapy		Physical Therapist	
265	Emergency Communications System		I. V. Therapy		Radiologic Technologist	
270	Trauma Treatment E. R.		Psychiatric Therapy		Dietetic Intern	
275	Orthopedic Emergency Services		Clinical Psychologist Services		Administration Residency	
280	Radioisotope Decontamination Room		Vocational Services		Medical Records Technologist	
285	Emergency Helicopter Service		Inhalation Therapy		Social Worker	
290			Hyperbaric Chamber Services		Paramedic Education	
295			Blood Collection and Processing			
280			Sheltered Workshop			
285			Pharmacy Unit Dose System			
290			Pharmacy IV Additive Program			

CODE
1 — Separately Organized, Staffed, and Equipped Unit of Hospital.
2 — Service Maintained in Hospital.
3 — Service Contracted but Hospital Based.
4 — Service Purchased from Outside Contractor and Not Hospital Based.
5 — Service Not Provided in Hospital but Shared with Another Hospital Under Contract.
6 — Service Not Available.
7 — Clinic Services are commonly provided in the emergency suite to non-emergency out-patients by hospital-based physicians or residents.
8 — Service Available Through but Not Billed by Hospital.
9 — Service Available, but Not Used During Reporting Cycle.

Blue Cross of California

EXHIBIT B

ADDRESSES WHERE HOSPITAL SERVICES

ARE PROVIDED

Individual hospitals should provide addresses.

EXHIBIT C

COMPENSATION RATES

    I. Inpatient Per Diem Rate

   II. Psychiatric Per Diem Rate*

  III. Outpatient Payment Rate

*Applicable where the primary diagnosis is a mental disorder or a chemical dependency regardless of where the Member is located in the hospital.

EXHIBIT D

PHYSICIAN SERVICES NOT INCLUDED IN

COMPENSATION PROVIDED IN SECTION 6.8

Individual hospitals should provide list of excluded services.

<u>EXHIBIT E</u>

UTILIZATION REVIEW PROCEDURES

I. INTRODUCTION

A. BLUE CROSS shall establish a Utilization Review program by
    contracting with _____ (Review
    Organization) to conduct Utilization Review as provided in Article
    VII. BLUE CROSS and the Review Organization shall establish and
    maintain review procedures and screening criteria which take into
    account locally professionally acceptable standards for quality
    medical care.

B. The Utilization Review process has two primary objectives:

    1. To assure that Hospital Services and Medical Services provided
        to members are Medically Necessary in an inpatient setting;
        and

    2. To assure that Hospital Services and Medical Services meet
        locally developed community standards for quality care and are
        provided at the appropriate level of care.

C. BLUE CROSS shall accept approval decisions made by the Review
    Organization regarding Medical Necessity as binding on BLUE CROSS.
    Denial decisions shall be subject to the appeal procedures
    provided in Article 7.5.

II. DEFINITIONS

The following definitions are in addition to any definitions provided
in Article II of this Agreement:

A. "Certification Form" means a document on which is stated the
    Review Organization's determinations regarding the Utilization
    Review performed pursuant to this Agreement.

B. "Working Day" means any day, Monday through Friday, excluding
    legal holidays.

C. "Review Coordinator" means a professionally qualified person who
    is competent to conduct initial review, data analysis and other
    functions involved in the Utilization Review performed pursuant
    to this Agreement.

- 1 -

D. "Physician Advisor" means a validly licensed physician who is employed by or on contract to a Review Organization to carry out Utilization Review.

E. "Norms" means numerical or statistical measures of observed performance of health care services derived from aggregated information related to the health care services provided to a statistically significant number of persons, as developed by the Review Organization.

F. "Screening Criteria" means those written guidelines adopted by the Review Organization pursuant to this Exhibit E.

III. RESPONSIBILITIES OF PARTICIPATING PHYSICIANS, PARTICIPATING HOSPITALS AND THE REVIEW ORGANIZATION

A. Responsibilities of the Review Organization

1. The Review Organization shall develop, update, and maintain screening Criteria which shall be subject to the review and approval of Blue Cross.

   a. Screening Criteria shall be developed for the purpose of making an initial determination whether an inpatient hospital admission or continued inpatient hospital stay is Medically Necessary.

   b. Screening Criteria shall be based on professional expertise, current professional literature, and cumulative information on health care services provided within the community to a statistically significant number of persons.

   c. Screening Criteria shall be developed to enable the Review Coordinator to select for review by the Physician Advisor only those cases which appear outside locally accepted professional norms.

2. The Review Organization shall utilize professionally qualified review personnel to perform the duties of Review Coordinators. Such Review Coordinators shall have authority to use the Screening Criteria to provide pre-admission authorization, admission approval and assign approved lengths of stay for Members' inpatient hospital admission and inpatient stay. A Review Coordinator shall have no authority to deny inpatient hospital admission or inpatient stay.

- 2 -

3. The Review Organization may deny an inpatient hospital admission and continued inpatient hospital stay but only by a Physician Advisor, after a review by the Physician Advisor of information contained in the member's medical record and after consultation with the Participating Physician. If the Participating Physician is unavailable for consultation with the Physician Advisor and available information is insufficient for approval of the inpatient hospital admission or continued inpatient hospital stay, the Physician Advisor shall deny the admission or stay subject to reconsideration and other appeal as provided in the Agreement.

4. The Review Organization shall respond to requests for pre-admission review by providing a determination by telephone within one (1) Working Day of such requests. A control number shall be given to the Participating Physician or his authorized representative and to the hospital to which the patient is scheduled to be admitted when the telephone determination is made.

5. The Review Organization shall provide written notification, on a Pre-Admission Form, of approved requests for pre-admission review within three (3) Working Days of the requests. Such notification shall be mailed to the Participating Physician and Participating Hospital.

6. The Review Organization shall respond to requests for reconsideration of denied pre-admission requests pursuant to Section 7.4, by making a redetermination and communicating the results to the Participating Physician by telephone within one (1) Working Day of the request and in writing within three (3) Working Days of the request.

7. The Review Organization shall conduct admission and concurrent review of all Members' inpatient hospital admissions and continued inpatient hospital stays.

8. The Review Coordinator shall use the Screening Criteria to establish review dates for approved inpatient hospital stays. Review dates shall be noted on the Member's Medical Record. If the Member continues to be an inpatient, an additional concurrent review shall be conducted on or before the noted review date, a redetermination made and, if appropriate, a new review date established pursuant to this section. This process shall continue until either the Member is discharged or the Physician Advisor determines that, based on available information from the Member's medical record and the Participating Physician, a continued inpatient hospital stay is not approved.

- 3 -

9. If the Physician Advisor determines, on the basis of available information obtained from the Member's Medical Record and the Participating Physician, that a continued inpatient hospital stay is not approved, the Review Organization shall notify the Participating Hospital, the Participating Physician and the Member or the Member's authorized representative in writing, on the Certification Form, within one (1) Working Day. Such notification shall include an explanation of the procedure for requesting reconsideration.

10. If reconsideration of a denied continued inpatient hospital stay is requested, the Review Organization shall reconsider the decision and communicate it to the Participating Hospital, Participating Physician and Member, in writing, within no more than two (2) Working Days of the request if the Member is an inpatient. Otherwise, the Review Organization shall notify the Participating Hospital, the Participating Physician and the Member or his authorized representative of the reconsideration decision, in writing, on the Certification Form, within twenty (20) Working Days of the request. Further appeal shall be conducted, if requested, according to the appeal procedures provided in Article 7.5.

11. In making any determination regarding whether an inpatient hospital admission or a continued inpatient hospital stay is Medically Necessary, the Review Organization shall consider all relevant information. The Review Organization shall thoroughly document its actions and the rationale for its determinations.

B. Responsibilities of the Participating Physician

1. To avoid retrospective denial of payment for inpatient services provided to Prudent Buyer Members, the Participating Physician shall request a pre-admission review from the Review Organization at least three (3) Working Days prior to a scheduled admission for inpatient admission for those diagnoses and procedures listed in Exhibit F, or for a scheduled referral to a non-participating hospital, as provided in V of this Exhibit E.

2. At least the following information shall be provided by the Participating Physician to the Review Organization at the time of the request for pre-authorization:

    a. Patient's name and identification number,
    b. Patient's age and sex,
    c. Diagnosis,
    d. Reason for admission,

- 4 -

e. Scheduled date of admission,
f. Planned procedure or surgery,
g. Date of planned procedure or surgery,
h. Name of hospital to which the member will be admitted,
i. Name and telephone of Participating Physician,
j. Other information as may be requested by the Review Organization.

C. Participating Hospital

1. If the Participating Hospital has not received notice of a pre-admission determination as required by this Agreement, at the time of a scheduled admission, it shall contact the Participating Physician or the Review Organization to request the determination. Any admission that requires pre-admission review pursuant to this Agreement and has not received that review, may be subject to retrospective denial. The information required for the pre-admission review shall be the same as provided in III.B.2. of this Exhibit E.

2. The Participating Hospital shall notify the Review Organization of the admission at the time the Member is admitted. If a Member is admitted on other than a Working Day, the Participating Hospital shall notify the Review Organization of the admission during the morning of the next Working Day following the admission.

IV. OTHER PROCEDURES AND INFORMATION

A. Utilization Review and Payment of Claims

1. The Certification Form shall be attached to the claim form when the claim form is submitted to Blue Cross for payment. Claim forms without the Certification Form attached will be returned to the Participating Provider.

2. Participating Providers submitting claims by way of electronic data entry shall indicate, in the appropriate space on the screen, that the Certification Form is on file with the Participating Provider. Claims without that indication will be rejected.

B. Responsibility for Payment Determination

The Utilization Review decision made by the Review Organization is solely for determining whether Hospital

Services and Medical Services are Medically Necessary in an
inpatient setting. Claim processing and payment determination shall be the sole responsibility of Blue Cross.

V. REFERRAL CARE

A. Scheduled Referral to Non-Participating Hospitals

1. Any scheduled referrals for Hospital Services or Medical
Services to non-participating hospitals require pre-
authorization review and approval by the Review Organization,
if the Member is to receive the maximum benefit available
under the Prudent Buyer Benefit Agreement.

2. Pre-admission review for referral care shall be requested by
the Participating Physician and shall be performed according
to this Exhibit E. The Review Organization shall determine
whether the services are Medically Necessary and whether they
could be provided at a Participating Hospital. The Review
Organization shall not authorize inpatient hospital admission
or continued inpatient hospital stays which could be provided
at a Participating Hospital in a manner consistent with the
needs of the Member.

3. The Review Organization shall provide notification of the
determination regarding referral care by telephone within one
(1) Working Day of the request for pre-admission review and
in writing, on the Certification Form, within three (3)
Working Days of the request.

B. Emergency admission to and continued hospital stay at non-
participating hospitals shall be reviewed by the Review
Organization to determine whether the stay is Medically Necessary
and whether the Member should be transferred for continued care
to a Participating Hospital in order to receive the maximum
benefits available under the Prudent Buyer Benefit Agreement.

VI. DELEGATION OF UTILIZATION REVIEW ACTIVITIES

Participating hospitals currently approved for delegated review for
their private patients by their Review Organization will be
considered as delegated for the Prudent Buyer Program.

Participating hospitals currently not approved for delegated review
for their private patients by their Review Organization will be
considered as non-delegated for the Prudent Buyer Program.

Participating hospitals with delegated status will be evaluated each
calendar quarter by the Review Organization. If the criteria for
delegation continues to be met, delegated status will be retained for
the following calendar quarter. However, if the criteria for
delegation is not met, delegated status will be withdrawn for the
following calendar quarter.

Participating hospitals without delegated status may request to be
evaluated for delegated status following one calendar quarter of
utilization activity which included at least 50 hospitals discharges
(excluding obstetrics).

Participating hospitals will be evaluated with the following
Structural Criteria and Procedural Criteria in order to both qualify
and maintain delegated status for concurrent review.

A. Structural Criteria

    1. Documentation that a Utilization Review Committee (U.R.C.) is
        formally constituted, organized and approved by the
        hospital's medical staff and governing body with the
        responsibility for the mechanisms needed to assure proper
        utilization of hospital services.

    2. Documentation that the U.R.C. includes (or plans to include)
        broad specialty representation of the medical staff.

    3. Documentation that the U.R. program insures (or has the
        capability to insure) that decisions on medical questions are
        made solely by the medical staff members.

    4. Documentation that the U.R.C. meets customarily, at least
        monthly, with regular attendance of members.

    5. Documentation that physicians do not have a vote in decisions
        concerning review of their own cases.

    6. Assurance that the U.R.C. and the U.R. program receives
        administrative support deemed necessary by the medical
        staff.

    7. Documentation that the hospital employes a U.R. Coordinator
        or identifies an employee who has responsibility for daily
        review coordination and communication with the Review
        Organization.

B. Procedural Criteria

   1. Ability for correct usage of intensity of services and levels
of care criteria. This includes the ability to reassess and
modify length-of-stay certifications according to current
information about an individual case.

   2. Ability for correct usage of Review Organization forms.

   3. Ability for correct usage of Review Organization's review
procedures for timeliness of reviews, advance notification,
appeal periods, extensions, and final notifications.

   4. Ability to provide the Review Organization with accurate and
timely statistical data on cases reviewed.

C. Measurement Criterion

   1. Participating hospitals will be evaluated with the following
Measurement Criterion to qualify for delegated status for
concurrent review:

     Less than 2.5% disagreement rate for approved cases vs. non-
approved cases between the Participating Hospital and the
Review Organization.

   2. Participating Hospitals will be evaluated with the following
Measurement Criterion to maintain delegated status for
concurrent review:

     Less than 2.5% disagreement rate for approved vs. non-
approved days of care between the Participating Hospital and
the Review Organization.

VII. PARTICIPATING PROVIDER COMMITTEE

A. A committee composed equally of Participating Hospitals and
Participating Physicians shall be appointed by the Blue Cross
Board of Directors by January 1, 1984. The Committee shall be
known as the Prudent Buyer Plan Participating Provider Committee
(Committee) and shall advise the Blue Cross Board of Directors
and Blue Cross staff on Utilization Review policies, procedures
and screening criteria as established and administered pursuant
to this Exhibit E, Exhibit F, and Article VII.

B. Until such time as the Committee is appointed, the Blue Cross of
California Physician Advisory Committee and Hospital Relations
Committee shall act in the Committee's place.

C. The Committee shall consist of twenty-six (26) Members. Twelve
    (12) participating physicians shall be appointed: One (1) each
    from among Participating Physicians nominated by the County
    Medical Societies in each of the Council Districts of the
    California Medical Association, with one (1) Participating
    Physician appointed from each California Medical Association
    Council District, and one additional physician shall be
    appointed from among Participating Physicians nominated by the
    medical staff organizations of Participating teaching
    hospitals.

    Twelve (12) representatives of Participating Hospitals shall be
    appointed. Four each shall be from among those nominated by the
    Hospital Council of Northern California and the Hospital Council
    of Southern California and two each shall be from among those
    nominated by the Hospital Council of Central California and the
    Hospital Council of San Diego and Imperial Counties.

    The Chairman and Vice Chairman of the Committee, one of whom
    shall be a Participating Physician and one of whom shall be a
    representative of a Participating Hospital, shall be appointed
    by the Blue Cross Board of Directors from among hospital
    representatives and physicians who are members of at least one
    of the following:

        The Blue Cross of California Board of Directors, the
        Blue Cross of Northern California Board of Directors,
        the Blue Cross of Southern California Board of Directors,
        the Blue Cross of California Physician Advisory Committee,
        or the Blue Cross of California Hospital Relations
        Committee.

    Appointments shall be for three year terms, with initial
    appointments staggered for one, two and three year appointments.

EXHIBIT F

DIAGNOSIS AND PROCEDURES
REQUIRING PREADMISSION REVIEW

The diagnosis and procedures listed below should receive preadmission review and authorization for guaranteed payment on inpatient hospitalization. They are divided into the following three categories:

Category I: Medical Necessity

Procedures always requiring prior authorization for the medical necessity of inpatient care.

Category II: Procedures Customarily Performed in an Ambulatory Setting

Procedures generally performed in an ambulatory setting which require prior authorization, based upon documentation of extra risk factors, for guaranteed payment of inpatient care.

Category III: May be Excluded as Inpatient Benefit in the Benefit Agreement

Diagnosis and procedures which may be excluded as contract benefits for inpatient care in the Blue Cross Benefit Agreement.

CATEGORY I: MEDICAL NECESSITY

1. Scheduled procedure or treatment requiring hospitalization but not due to be performed within twenty-four (24) hours of admission

2. Non-emergency psychiatric admissions

3. Bunionectomy

4. Frenulectomy

5. Gynecomastia excision

6. Hammertoe repair with tenotomies and resection of bone

7. Submucous resection of nasal septum

8. Chemical dependency admissions

CATEGORY II: PROCEDURES CUSTOMARILY PERFORMED IN AN AMBULATORY SETTING

1. Integumentary System

    Breast biopsy - incision, excision (uni or bilateral)
    Excision of sebaceous cyst
    Mandible cyst excision - simple
    Pilonidal cyst excision, simple
    Simple excision, lymph node
    Skin graft, small
    Treatment of condylomata acuminate (male/female)

2. Musculoskeletal System

    Arthrodesis, fingers or toes
    Arthroplasty, small joints
    Arthroscopy of the knee where definitive procedure not planned
    Arthrotomy, small joint
    Bone marrow biopsy
    Bursectomy (simple)
    Capsulectomy/Capsulotomy, small joints
    Chondroplasty by arthroscopy
    Chronic pain evaluation plus rehabilitation
    Foreign body removal, superficial
    Fusion of small joints (i.e., interphalangeal)
    Ganglionectomy
    Joint manipulation
    Muscle biopsy
    Neuroma excision (Mortons and cutaneous and digital nerves)
    Ostectomy metatarsal (metatarsal head excision)
    Osteotomy
    Phalangectomy, partial or total
    Scar revision
    Simple exostosectomy of small bones
    Surgical aftercare, superficial wire removal, extremity
    Synovectomy - simple
    Tendon sheath release (De Quervains)
    Tenotomy hands, fingers, ankles, feet and toes
    Trigger finger release
    Zygoma (Zygomatic arch) reduction (simple)

3. Respiratory System

    Bronchoscopy
    Laryngoscopy as an only procedure

4. Cardiovascular System

    Routine cardiovascular non-invasive diagnostic procedures
    Temporal artery, ligation or biopsy
    Varicose vein ligation

5. Digestive System

    Branchial arch appendage excision (simple)
    Colostomy revision (simple)
    Fistulectomy (small)
    Gastrointestinal endoscopy (uncomplicated)
    Liver biopsy, percutaneous
    Paracentesis
    Rectal polypectomy (simple)
    Sigmoidoscopy
    Wedge resection of lip

6. Urinary System

    Cystoscopy
    Meatotomy
    Urethral dilatation

7. Male Genital System

    Circumcision
    Hydrocele excision
    Prostate biopsy, needle
    Vasectomy

8. Female Genital System

    Abortion, Therapeutic (1st trimester)
    Biopsy of cervix, endometrium, (endometrial aspiration or washing), vagina
    Cauterization of cervix
    Circumferential conization
    Cryotherapy with biopsy and/or endocervical curettage
    Culdoscopy (culdocentesis)
    Dilatation and curettage (diagnositc or therapeutic)
    Fulguration, vulva and cervix
    Hymenotomy
    Hysterosalpinogram
    Laparoscopy
    Pelvic exam under anesthesia
    Removal of IUD
    Tubal ligation
    Use of laser in treating lesions of cervix, vagina or vulva
    Vaginal stenosis release (simple)
    Vaginal-tumor (cyst) excision
    Vulva (labial) biopsy

9. Nervous System

    Decompression of the Medial Nerve at the Carpal Tunnel
    Nerve biopsy
    Nerve block
    Nerve repair, simple
    Neurectomy
    Neurolysis, simple

- 4 -

10. <u>Eye and Ocular Adnexa System</u>

   Cataract excision by phako-emulsification with/without implant
   Chalazion excision
   Discission lens (needling of lens)
   Ectropion/entropion repair
   Foreign body removal
   Lacrimal duct probing
   Pterygium (excision or transposition)
   Tarsorrhaphy

11. <u>Otorhinolaryngology (Ear, Nose, Throat)</u>

   Antral puncture
   Resection of turbinate
   Inferior turbinate fracture
   Myringoplasty
   Nasal polypectomy (small or few)
   Nose, closed reduction
   Otoscopy, with or without removal of foreign body
   Tongue biopsy

CATEGORY III: MAY BE EXCLUDED AS INPATIENT BENEFIT

The following diagnosis and procedures are generally excluded from Blue Cross Benefit Agreements:

1. Allergy and environmental control

2. Behavior problems

3. Blepharoplasty (upper, lower or combined)

4. Chelation therapy for other than acute metal toxicity (e.g., ASHD)

5. Cosmetic or reconstructive surgery -- all types

6. Developmental problem(s)

7. Eating disorder(s)

8. Facial dermabrasion

9. Learning disability(ies)

10. Mammoplasty (augmentation)

11. Obesity

12. Otoplasty (unilateral/bilateral)

13. Rhytidectomy

14. Vermilionectomy

Blue Cross of California

EXHIBIT G

ARBITRATION FOR UTILIZATION REVIEW

The initial decision regarding whether Hospital Services or Medical Services are Medically Necessary shall be made pursuant to Section 7.2. HOSPITAL may appeal such a decision pursuant to the terms of Section 7.5. Arbitration under that section shall follow the procedures below:

A. HOSPITAL, agrees to submit any dispute concerning a Utilization Review decision, unresolved by reconsideration or review pursuant to the terms of Section 7.2, to binding arbitration. The arbitration shall be commenced by HOSPITAL making written demand on BLUE CROSS. The scope of that arbitration shall be limited to a determination of whether, or to what extent, benefits specified in the applicable Prudent Buyer Benefit Agreement were Medically Necessary or otherwise payable for the claim or claims in dispute.

B. The arbitration shall be held before a neutral arbitrator appointed by the county medical association of the county in which the services were provided. If the county medical association declines or is unable to appoint an arbitrator, the arbitrator shall be appointed by the superior court having jurisdiction over the matter according to California Code of Civil Procedure Section 1281.6, or as otherwise mutually agreed in writing by BLUE CROSS and HOSPITAL.

C. Any arbitration shall be conducted according to the California Arbitration Act, Code of Civil Procedure Section 1280 et seq., or as otherwise mutually agreed. HOSPITAL and BLUE CROSS agree that the arbitration findings shall be binding upon any subsequent litigation.

APPENDIX C

Blue Cross of California Participating Physician Agreement*

*The material in this section related to sample contracts appears with the cooperation and permission of the Blue Cross of California. We thank that organization for its help in making this available.

BLUE CROSS OF CALIFORNIA

PARTICIPATING PHYSICIAN AGREEMENT

TABLE OF CONTENTS

EXHIBITS

BLUE CROSS OF CALIFORNIA

PARTICIPATING PHYSICIAN AGREEMENT

This AGREEMENT is effective on _____, 1983, between BLUE CROSS OF
CALIFORNIA ("BLUE CROSS") and _____
("PHYSICIAN").

I. RECITALS

1.1 BLUE CROSS is a California non-profit hospital service corporation,
     duly licensed by the Insurance Commissioner of the State of California,
     pursuant to Insurance Code Section 11495 et seq., to issue benefit
     agreements covering the provision of health care services and to enter
     into agreements with PHYSICIAN.

1.2 PHYSICIAN is a "licensee" as that term is defined under Business and
     Professions Code Section 2041.

1.3 BLUE CROSS intends by entering into this Agreement to make available
     quality health care to Blue Cross Prudent Buyer Members by contracting
     with PHYSICIAN. PHYSICIAN intends to provide such quality health care
     in a cost-efficient manner.

II. DEFINITIONS

2.1 "Benefit Agreement(s)" means the written agreement entered into by
     BLUE CROSS and groups or individuals under which BLUE CROSS provides,
     indemnifies, or administers health care benefits.

2.2 "Emergency" means a sudden onset of a medical condition manifesting
     itself by acute symptoms of sufficient severity that the absence of
     immediate medical attention could reasonably result in:

        (1) permanently placing the Member's health in jeopardy,

        (2) causing other serious medical consequences,

- 1 -

      (3)   causing serious impairment to bodily functions, or

      (4)   causing serious and permanent dysfunction of any bodily organ or part.

2.3   "Hospital Services" means those acute care inpatient and hospital outpatient services which are covered by a Prudent Buyer Benefit Agreement. Hospital Services do not include long-term non-acute care.

2.4   "Medically Necessary" means services or supplies which, under the provisions of this Agreement, are determined to be:

      (1)   Appropriate and necessary for the symptoms, diagnosis or treatment of the medical condition, and

      (2)   Provided for the diagnosis or direct care and treatment of the medical condition, and

      (3)   Within standards of good medical practice within the organized medical community, and

      (4)   Not primarily for the convenience of the Member, the Member's physician or another provider, and

      (5)   The most appropriate supply or level of service which can safely be provided. For hospital stays, this means that acute care as an inpatient is necessary due to the kind of services the Member is receiving or the severity of the Member's condition, and that safe and adequate care cannot be received as an outpatient or in a less intensified medical setting.

2.5   "Medical Services" means those services provided by a Participating Physician and covered by a Prudent Buyer Benefit Agreement.

2.6   "Member(s)" means Subscribers or enrolled dependents covered by a Prudent Buyer Benefit Agreement.

2.7   "Prudent Buyer Benefit Agreement" means a Benefit Agreement pursuant to which Members have a financial incentive to use Participating Providers.

2.8   "Participating Hospital" means a hospital which has entered into an agreement to provide Hospital Services as a Participating Provider.

2.9   "Participating Physician" means a physician who has entered into an agreement to provide Medical Services as a Participating Provider and who is a "licensee" as that term is defined in Business and Professions Section 2041.

2.10 "Participating Provider" means a hospital, other health facility, physician or other health professional which has entered into an agreement with BLUE CROSS to provide health care services for prospectively determined rates.

2.11 "Subscribers" means individuals who have qualified for and are covered by the provisions of a Prudent Buyer Benefit Agreement.

2.12 "Utilization Review" means a function performed by an organization or entity acting as an agent of BLUE CROSS, and selected by BLUE CROSS to review and approve whether Medical Services provided, or to be provided, are Medically Necessary.

III. RELATIONSHIP BETWEEN BLUE CROSS AND PHYSICIAN

3.1   BLUE CROSS and PHYSICIAN are independent entities. Nothing in this Agreement shall be construed or be deemed to create a relationship of employer and employee or principal and agent or any relationship other than that of independent parties contracting with each other solely for the purpose of carrying out the provisions of this Agreement.

3.2   BLUE CROSS and PHYSICIAN agree that PHYSICIAN shall maintain a physician/patient relationship with each Member that PHYSICIAN treats. PHYSICIAN shall be responsible solely to that Member for treatment and medical care.

3.3   Nothing in this Agreement is intended to be construed, or be deemed to create any rights or remedies in any third party, including but not limited to a Member or a Participating Provider other than PHYSICIAN.

IV. PHYSICIAN SERVICES AND RESPONSIBILITIES

4.1   PHYSICIAN shall provide to Members Medical Services which are Medically Necessary and which are in accordance with the applicable Prudent Buyer Benefit Agreement and this Agreement.

4.2   PHYSICIAN shall, to the extent possible, seek, accept and maintain evidence of assignment for the payment of Medical Services provided to Members by PHYSICIAN under the applicable Prudent Buyer Benefit Agreement.

4.3   PHYSICIAN agrees to admit or arrange for admission of Members only to Participating Hospitals unless otherwise determined by PHYSICIAN and agreed to by the Member. In case of an Emergency, as that term is defined in this Agreement, PHYSICIAN agrees to use a Participating Hospital whenever possible. Other exceptions to the use of Participating Hospitals shall be approved pursuant to the provisions of Article VII.

4.4   PHYSICIAN agrees to refer Members to other Participating Providers unless otherwise determined by PHYSICIAN and agreed to by the Member.

4.5   PHYSICIAN agrees to participate in the Utilization Review provided in Article VII and to abide by decisions resulting from that review subject to rights of reconsideration, review and arbitration provided in Section 7.5.

4.6   PHYSICIAN has accurately completed the Participating Physician Application which is attached to and made part of this Agreement as Exhibit A. PHYSICIAN shall promptly notify BLUE CROSS of any change in the information contained on the Application, including any change in its principal place of business, within thirty (30) days of such change.

V. BLUE CROSS SERVICES AND RESPONSIBILITIES

5.1   BLUE CROSS agrees to pay PHYSICIAN compensation pursuant to the provisions of Article VI.

5.2   BLUE CROSS agrees to grant PHYSICIAN the status of "Participating Physician", to identify PHYSICIAN as a Participating Physician on informational materials to Members, and to direct such Members to PHYSICIANS.

5.3   BLUE CROSS agrees to continue listing PHYSICIAN as a Participating Physician until this Agreement terminates pursuant to this Agreement.

5.4   BLUE CROSS agrees to provide PHYSICIAN with a list of all Participating Physicians, Participating Hospitals and other Participating Providers.

5.5   BLUE CROSS agrees to provide appropriate identification cards for Members.

5.6   Blue Cross agrees that the definitions of "Emergency" in Section 2.2 and "Medically Necessary" in Section 2.4 of the Prudent Buyer benefit agreements described in Section 2.1 and this agreement shall be consistent.

VI.   COMPENSATION AND BILLING

6.1   PHYSICIAN shall seek payment only from BLUE CROSS for the provision of Medical Services except as provided in Section 6.2. The payment from BLUE CROSS shall be limited to the amounts referred to in Section 6.6, less copayments and deductible amounts as provided in Section 6.5.

6.2   PHYSICIAN may also seek payment for the provision of Medical Services from other sources as provided in Section 6.3, and as available pursuant to the coordination of benefit provisions of the applicable Prudent Buyer Benefit Agreement and Section 6.4.

6.3   PHYSICIAN agrees that the only charges for which a Member may be liable and be billed by PHYSICIAN shall be for Medical Services not covered by the applicable Prudent Buyer Benefit Agreement, for copayments and deductible amounts required by the applicable Prudent Buyer Benefit Agreement, or as provided in Section 6.10.

6.4   In a case in which BLUE CROSS, under the applicable Prudent Buyer Benefit Agreement, is primary under applicable coordination of benefit rules provided in Title 10 of the California Administrative Code Sections 2232.50 through 2232.56, BLUE CROSS shall pay the amounts due under this Agreement reduced as provided in Section 6.5. In a case in which BLUE CROSS is other than primary under the coordination of benefit rules referred to above, BLUE CROSS shall pay only those amounts which when added to amounts received by PHYSICIAN from other sources pursuant to the applicable coordination of benefit rules, equals one hundred percent of the amounts required by this Agreement.

6.5   BLUE CROSS shall deduct any copayments and deductible amounts required by the applicable Prudent Buyer Benefit Agreement from payment due PHYSICIAN from BLUE CROSS pursuant to this Agreement.

6.6   PHYSICIAN agrees to accept the fee schedule as provided in Exhibit B, attached to and made part of this Agreement or PHYSICIAN'S billed charges, whichever is less, as payment in full for all Medical Services provided to Members. Such payment shall be for Medical Services provided on or after the effective date of this Agreement.
Should the fee schedule be less than the Medicare payment for the specific medical services, then the Medicare payment rate shall apply.

6.7   Prior to April 1 of each year, BLUE CROSS shall publish a fee schedule which shall be effective on the following August 1. The fee schedule shall be reviewed for comment by the Blue Cross Physician Advisory Committee prior to adoption.

6.8   PHYSICIAN shall bill BLUE CROSS on forms and in a manner acceptable to BLUE CROSS within twelve (12) months of performing the Medical Services. PHYSICIAN shall furnish, on request, all information reasonably required by BLUE CROSS to verify and substantiate the provision of Medical Services and the charges for such services. BLUE CROSS reserves the right to review all such information submitted by PHYSICIAN when necessary and in accordance with this Agreement.

6.9   BLUE CROSS shall pay PHYSICIAN within thirty (30) days of receipt of billings which are accurate, complete and otherwise in accordance with Section 6.8.

6.10   PHYSICIAN shall not charge Members for Medical Services denied as not being Medically Necessary under Section 7.2, unless the Member has agreed in writing to be responsible for payment of those charges. That agreement may be obtained by a Participating Hospital where the Member is an inpatient, on a form approved by BLUE Cross.

VII. UTILIZATION REVIEW

7.1   BLUE CROSS shall establish a Utilization Review program which shall seek to assure that Hospital Services and Medical Services provided to Members are Medically Necessary in an inpatient setting. The Utilization Review shall follow the procedures provided on Exhibit C, attached to and made part of this Agreement.

7.2   Utilization Review for inpatient Medical Services shall include:

1)   "Pre-admission review" to determine whether a scheduled inpatient admission is Medically Necessary. Pre-admission review procedures are provided in Exhibit D, attached to and made part of this Agreement.

2)   "Admission review" to determine whether an unscheduled inpatient admission or an admission not subject to pre-admission review is Medically Necessary.

3)   "Concurrent review" to determine whether a continued inpatient hospital stay is Medically Necessary.

7.3   BLUE CROSS shall conduct retrospective review to determine whether
outpatient services were Medically Necessary. Any appeal of a decision
under this Section shall be commenced by requesting a review by BLUE
CROSS. If not satisfied, PHYSICIAN may request arbitration as provided
in Exhibit E, attached to and made part of this Agreement.

7.4   Blue Cross shall not retrospectively deny any inpatient services
approved under Section 7.2.

7.5   PHYSICIAN may appeal a Utilization Review decision. The appeal shall
be commenced by requesting reconsideration by the organization or
entity making the initial decision. If PHYSICIAN is not satisfied with
that result, it may request a review by BLUE CROSS. If PHYSICIAN
continues not to be satisfied, it may request arbitration as provided
in Exhibit E.

VIII. RECORDS MAINTENANCE, AVAILABILITY, INSPECTION AND AUDIT

8.1   PHYSICIAN agrees to allow review and duplication of any
data and other records maintained on Members which relate to
this Agreement. Medical records shall be made available as necessary
for provision of Medical Services and as otherwise necessary to carry
out the terms of this Agreement. Such availability, review and
duplication shall be allowed upon reasonable notice during regular
business hours and shall be subject to all applicable laws and
regulations concerning the confidentiality of such data or records.

8.2   Ownership and access to records of Members shall be controlled by
applicable law.

IX. LIABILITY,INDEMNITY AND INSURANCE

9.1   Neither BLUE CROSS nor PHYSICIAN nor any of their respective agents or
employees shall be liable to third parties for any act or omission of
the other party.

9.2   PHYSICIAN, at its sole expense, agrees to maintain adequate insurance
for professional liability and comprehensive general liability.
In lieu of any insurance required by this section, PHYSICIAN shall
maintain the ability to respond to any and all damages which would be
covered by such insurance.

9.3   Upon request by BLUE CROSS, PHYSICIAN shall provide BLUE CROSS
with copies of insurance policies or evidence of the ability to respond
to any and all damages as provided in Section 9.2.

X. MARKETING, ADVERTISING AND PUBLICITY

   10.1 BLUE CROSS shall use its best efforts to encourage Members to use the
         services of PHYSICIAN.

   10.2 BLUE CROSS shall have the right to use the name of PHYSICIAN for
         purposes of informing Members and prospective Members of the identity
         of Participating Physicians. The materials using the name of PHYSICIAN
         shall be reviewed by the BLUE CROSS Physician Advisory Committee prior
         to use.

   10.3 Except as provided in Section 10.2, BLUE CROSS and PHYSICIAN each
         reserves the right to and the control of the use of its name and all
         symbols, trademarks or service marks presently existing or later
         established. In addition, except as provided in Section 10.2, neither
         BLUE CROSS nor PHYSICIAN shall use the other party's name, symbols,
         trademarks or service marks in advertising or promotional materials
         or otherwise without the prior written consent of that party and shall
         cease any such usage immediately upon written notice of the party or
         on termination of this Agreement, whichever is sooner.

XI. DISPUTE RESOLUTION

   11.1 BLUE CROSS and PHYSICIAN agree to meet and confer in good faith to
         resolve any problems or disputes that may arise under this Agreement.

   11.2 In the event that any problem or dispute concerning the terms of this
         Agreement, other than a Utilization Review decision as provided for
         in Article VII, is not satisfactorily resolved, BLUE CROSS and
         PHYSICIAN agree to arbitrate such problem or dispute. Such arbitration
         shall be initiated by either party making a written demand for
         arbitration on the other party. Within thirty (30) days of that
         demand, BLUE CROSS and PHYSICIAN shall each designate an arbitrator
         and give written notice of such designation to the other. Within
         thirty (30) days after these notices have been given, the two
         arbitrators selected by this process shall select a third neutral
         arbitrator and give notice of the selection to BLUE CROSS and
         PHYSICIAN. The three arbitrators shall hold a hearing and decide
         the matter within sixty (60) days thereafter.

   11.3 The arbitration shall be conducted pursuant to the California Code
         of Civil Procedure, Title Nine, Section 1280, et seq., unless otherwise
         mutually agreed. PHYSICIAN and BLUE CROSS agree that the arbitration
         results shall be binding on both parties in any subsequent litigation
         or other dispute.

XII. TERM AND TERMINATION

12.1　When executed by both parties, this Agreement shall become effective as of the date noted on page 1 and shall continue in effect until terminated pursuant to this Agreement.

12.2　Either party may terminate this Agreement, by giving at least ninety (90) days' prior written notice. Nothing contained herein shall be construed to limit either party's lawful remedies in the event of a material breach of this Agreement.

12.3　Notwithstanding termination, BLUE CROSS shall continue to have access to records for four (4) years from the date of provision of the Medical services to which the records refer. Such records shall available in accordance with Article VIII, to the extent permitted by law and as necessary to fulfill the terms of this Agreement.

12.4　After the effective date of termination, this Agreement shall remain in effect for the resolution of all matters unresolved at that date.

XIII. GENERAL PROVISIONS

13.1　Assignment

No assignment of the rights, duties, or obligations of this Agreement shall be made by PHYSICIAN without the express written approval of a duly authorized representative of BLUE CROSS. Any attempted assignment in violation of this provision shall be void as to BLUE CROSS.

13.2　Waiver of Breach

Waiver of a breach of any provision of this Agreement shall not be deemed a waiver of any other breach of the same or different provision.

13.3　Notices

Any notice required to be given pursuant to the terms and provisions of this Agreement shall be in writing, postage prepaid, and shall be sent by certified mail, return receipt requested, to BLUE CROSS or PHYSICIAN at the addresses below. The notice shall be effective on the date indicated on the return receipt.

Provider Contracting Department
Nineteenth Floor
Blue Cross of California
1950 Franklin Street
Oakland, California 94659

and to PHYSICIAN at:

13.4 Severability

In the event any provision of this Agreement is rendered invalid or
unenforceable by an Act of Congress or of the California Legislature or
by any regulation duly promulgated by officers of the United States or
of the State of California acting in accordance with law, or declared
null and void by any court of competent jurisdiction, the remainder of
the provisions of this Agreement shall, subject to paragraph 13.5,
remain in full force and effect.

13.5 Effect of Severable Provision

In the event that a provision of this Agreement is rendered invalid or
unenforceable or declared null and void as provided in Section 13.4 and
its removal has the effect of materially altering the obligations of
either party in such manner as, in the judgment of the party affected,
(a) will cause serious financial hardship to such party; or (b) will
cause such party to act in violation of its corporate Articles or
Bylaws, the party so affected shall have the right to terminate this
Agreement upon thirty (30) days' prior written notice to the other
party.   The applicable provisions of Article XII shall apply to such
termination.

13.6 Entire Agreement

This Agreement, together with exhibits, contains the entire Agreement
between BLUE CROSS and PHYSICIAN relating to the rights granted and the
obligations assumed by this Agreement. Any prior agreements, promises,
negotiations or representations, either oral or written, relating to
the subject matter of this Agreement not expressly set forth in this
Agreement are of no force or effect.

13.7 Amendment

This Agreement or any article or section of it may be amended at
any time during the term of the Agreement by mutual written consent of
duly authorized representatives of the parties.

13.8 Attorneys' Fees

In the event that either BLUE CROSS or PHYSICIAN institutes any action,
suit, or arbitration proceeding to enforce the provisions of this
Agreement, each party shall pay one half of the arbitration costs and
otherwise pay its own attorneys' fees and other costs.

13.9 Headings

The headings of articles and sections contained in this Agreement
are for reference purposes only and shall not affect in any way the
meaning or interpretation of this Agreement.

13.10 Governing Law

This Agreement shall be construed and enforced in accordance with the
laws of the State of California.

FOR BLUE CROSS   FOR PHYSICIAN

_____   _____

Title:_____   Title:_____

Date:_____   Date:_____

BLUE CROSS OF CALIFORNIA

EXHIBIT A

PARTICIPATING PHYSICIAN APPLICATION

Last name	First name		Initial

Office stree address (Primary location	City	State	Zip	Telephone

(Additional locations)		Telephone

Mailing address	City	State	Zip

Tax Identification #	License #	Social Security #

If not in solo practice, indicate name of group and/or nature of affiliation:

_____

Has your license to practice medicine in any jurisdiction ever been revoked, suspended, or subject to probation? _____ If yes, please attach explanation.

MEDICAL SPECIALTY

Specialty: Primary_____ Secondary_____

Practice limited to: _____

ESTIMATED CAPACITY

In my practice, I can comfortably see _____ patients per day.

Estimated capacity for additional patients:

For primary care physician, _____ additional patients.

For specialist, _____ additional patients per month.

HOSPITAL STAFF PRIVILEGES

List all hospitals in which you have admitting privileges:

_____

_____

Signed: _____

Date:. _____

EXHIBIT C

UTILIZATION REVIEW PROCEDURES

I.   INTRODUCTION

   A.   BLUE CROSS shall establish a Utilization Review program by
        contracting with _____ (Review
        Organization) to conduct Utilization Review as provided in Article
        VII. BLUE CROSS and the Review Organization shall establish and
        maintain review procedures and screening criteria which take into
        account locally professionally acceptable standards for quality
        medical care.

   B.   The Utilization Review process has two primary objectives:

        1.   To assure that Hospital Services and Medical Services provided
             to members are Medically Necessary in an inpatient setting;
             and

        2.   To assure that Hospital Services and Medical Services meet
             locally developed community standards for quality care and are
             provided at the appropriate level of care.

   C.   BLUE CROSS shall accept approval decisions made by the Review
        Organization regarding Medical Necessity as binding on BLUE CROSS.
        Denial decisions shall be subject to the appeal procedures
        provided in Article 7.5.

II. DEFINITIONS

   The following definitions are in addition to any definitions provided
   in Article II of this Agreement:

   A.   "Certification Form" means a document on which is stated the
        Review Organization's determinations regarding the Utilization
        Review performed pursuant to this Agreement.

   B.   "Working Day" means any day, Monday through Friday, excluding
        legal holidays.

   C.   "Review Coordinator" means a professionally qualified person who
        is competent to conduct initial review, data analysis and other
        functions involved in the Utilization Review performed pursuant
        to this Agreement.

- 1 -

D. "Physician Advisor" means a validly licensed physician who is
    employed by or on contract to a Review Organization to carry out
    Utilization Review.

E. "Norms" means numerical or statistical measures of observed
    performance of health care services derived from aggregated
    information related to the health care services provided to a
    statistically significant number of persons, as developed by the
    Review Organization.

F. "Screening Criteria" means those written guidelines adopted by
    the Review Organization pursuant to this Exhibit E.

III. RESPONSIBILITIES OF PARTICIPATING PHYSICIANS, PARTICIPATING
      HOSPITALS AND THE REVIEW ORGANIZATION

A. Responsibilities of the Review Organization

    1. The Review Organization shall develop, update, and maintain
        screening Criteria which shall be subject to the review and
        approval of Blue Cross.

        a. Screening Criteria shall be developed for the purpose of
            making an initial determination whether an inpatient
            hospital admission or continued inpatient hospital stay
            is Medically Necessary.

        b. Screening Criteria shall be based on professional
            expertise, current professional literature, and
            cumulative information on health care services provided
            within the community to a statistically significant
            number of persons.

        c. Screening Criteria shall be developed to enable the
            Review Coordinator to select for review by the Physician
            Advisor only those cases which appear outside locally
            accepted professional norms.

    2. The Review Organization shall utilize professionally
        qualified review personnel to perform the duties of Review
        Coordinators. Such Review Coordinators shall have
        authority to use the Screening Criteria to provide pre-
        admission authorization, admission approval and assign
        approved lengths of stay for Members' inpatient hospital
        admission and inpatient stay. A Review Coordinator shall
        have no authority to deny inpatient hospital admission or
        inpatient stay.

- 2 -

3. The Review Organization may deny an inpatient hospital admission and continued inpatient hospital stay but only by a Physician Advisor, after a review by the Physician Advisor of information contained in the member's medical record and after consultation with the Participating Physician. If the Participating Physician is unavailable for consultation with the Physician Advisor and available information is insufficient for approval of the inpatient hospital admission or continued inpatient hospital stay, the Physician Advisor shall deny the admission or stay subject to reconsideration and other appeal as provided in the Agreement.

4. The Review Organization shall respond to requests for pre-admission review by providing a determination by telephone within one (1) Working Day of such requests. A control number shall be given to the Participating Physician or his authorized representative and to the hospital to which the patient is scheduled to be admitted when the telephone determination is made.

5. The Review Organization shall provide written notification, on a Pre-Admission Form, of approved requests for pre-admission review within three (3) Working Days of the requests. Such notification shall be mailed to the Participating Physician and Participating Hospital.

6. The Review Organization shall respond to requests for reconsideration of denied pre-admission requests pursuant to Section 7.4, by making a redetermination and communicating the results to the Participating Physician by telephone within one (1) Working Day of the request and in writing within three (3) Working Days of the request.

7. The Review Organization shall conduct admission and concurrent review of all Members' inpatient hospital admissions and continued inpatient hospital stays.

8. The Review Coordinator shall use the Screening Criteria to establish review dates for approved inpatient hospital stays. Review dates shall be noted on the Member's Medical Record. If the Member continues to be an inpatient, an additional concurrent review shall be conducted on or before the noted review date, a redetermination made and, if appropriate, a new review date established pursuant to this section. This process shall continue until either the Member is discharged or the Physician Advisor determines that, based on available information from the Member's medical record and the Participating Physician, a continued inpatient hospital stay is not approved.

- 3 -

9. If the Physician Advisor determines, on the basis of
    available information obtained from the Member's Medical
    Record and the Participating Physician, that a continued
    inpatient hospital stay is not approved, the Review
    Organization shall notify the Participating Hospital, the
    Participating Physician and the Member or the Member's
    authorized representative in writing, on the Certification
    Form, within one (1) Working Day. Such notification shall
    include an explanation of the procedure for requesting
    reconsideration.

10. If reconsideration of a denied continued inpatient hospital
    stay is requested, the Review Organization shall reconsider
    the decision and communicate it to the Participating
    Hospital, Participating Physician and Member, in writing,
    within no more than two (2) Working Days of the request if
    the Member is an inpatient. Otherwise, the Review
    Organization shall notify the Participating Hospital, the
    Participating Physician and the Member or his authorized
    representative of the reconsideration decision, in writing,
    on the Certification Form, within twenty (20) Working Days
    of the request. Further appeal shall be conducted, if
    requested, according to the appeal procedures provided in
    Article 7.5.

11. In making any determination regarding whether an inpatient
    hospital admission or a continued inpatient hospital stay
    is Medically Necessary, the Review Organization shall
    consider all relevant information. The Review Organization
    shall thoroughly document its actions and the rationale for
    its determinations.

B. Responsibilities of the Participating Physician

1. To avoid retrospective denial of payment for inpatient
    services provided to Prudent Buyer Members, the
    Participating Physician shall request a pre-admission
    review from the Review Organization at least three (3)
    Working Days prior to a scheduled admission for inpatient
    admission for those diagnoses and procedures listed in
    Exhibit D, or for a scheduled referral to a non-partici-
    pating hospital, as provided in V of this Exhibit C.

2. At least the following information shall be provided by the
    Participating Physician to the Review Organization at the
    time of the request for pre-authorization:

    a. Patient's name and identification number,
    b. Patient's age and sex,
    c. Diagnosis,
    d. Reason for admission,

      e. Scheduled date of admission,
      f. Planned procedure or surgery,
      g. Date of planned procedure or surgery,
      h. Name of hospital to which the member will be admitted,
      i. Name and telephone of Participating Physician,
      j. Other information as may be requested by the Review Organization.

C. Participating Hospital

  1. If the Participating Hospital has not received notice of a pre-admission determination as required by this Agreement, at the time of a scheduled admission, it shall contact the Participating Physician or the Review Organization to request the determination. Any admission that requires pre-admission review pursuant to this Agreement and has not received that review, may be subject to retrospective denial. The information required for the pre-admission review shall be the same as provided in III.B.2. of this Exhibit C.

  2. The Participating Hospital shall notify the Review Organization of the admission at the time the Member is admitted. If a Member is admitted on other than a Working Day, the Participating Hospital shall notify the Review Organization of the admission during the morning of the next Working Day following the admission.

IV. OTHER PROCEDURES AND INFORMATION

A. Utilization Review and Payment of Claims

  1. The Certification Form shall be attached to the claim form when the claim form is submitted to Blue Cross for payment. Claim forms without the Certification Form attached will be returned to the Participating Provider.

  2. Participating Providers submitting claims by way of electronic data entry shall indicate, in the appropriate space on the screen, that the Certification Form is on file with the Participating Provider. Claims without that indication will be rejected.

B. Responsibility for Payment Determination

The Utilization Review decision made by the Review Organization is solely for determining whether Hospital

Services and Medical Services are Medically Necessary in an inpatient setting. Claim processing and payment determination shall be the sole responsibility of Blue Cross.

V. REFERRAL CARE

A. Scheduled Referral to Non-Participating Hospitals

1. Any scheduled referrals for Hospital Services or Medical Services to non-participating hospitals require pre-authorization review and approval by the Review Organization, if the Member is to receive the maximum benefit available under the Prudent Buyer Benefit Agreement.

2. Pre-admission review for referral care shall be requested by the Participating Physician and shall be performed according to this Exhibit C. The Review Organization shall determine whether the services are Medically Necessary and whether they could be provided at a Participating Hospital. The Review Organization shall not authorize inpatient hospital admission or continued inpatient hospital stays which could be provided at a Participating Hospital in a manner consistent with the needs of the Member.

3. The Review Organization shall provide notification of the determination regarding referral care by telephone within one (1) Working Day of the request for pre-admission review and in writing, on the Certification Form, within three (3) Working Days of the request.

B. Emergency admission to and continued hospital stay at non-participating hospitals shall be reviewed by the Review Organization to determine whether the stay is Medically Necessary and whether the Member should be transferred for continued care to a Participating Hospital in order to receive the maximum benefits available under the Prudent Buyer Benefit Agreement.

VI. DELEGATION OF UTILIZATION REVIEW ACTIVITIES

Participating hospitals currently approved for delegated review for their private patients by their Review Organization will be considered as delegated for the Prudent Buyer Program.

Participating hospitals currently not approved for delegated review for their private patients by their Review Organization will be considered as non-delegated for the Prudent Buyer Program.

Participating hospitals with delegated status will be evaluated each calendar quarter by the Review Organization. If the criteria for delegation continues to be met, delegated status will be retained for the following calendar quarter. However, if the criteria for delegation is not met, delegated status will be withdrawn for the following calendar quarter.

Participating hospitals without delegated status may request to be evaluated for delegated status following one calendar quarter of utilization activity which included at least 50 hospitals discharges (excluding obstetrics).

Participating hospitals will be evaluated with the following Structural Criteria and Procedural Criteria in order to both qualify and maintain delegated status for concurrent review.

A. Structural Criteria

1. Documentation that a Utilization Review Committee (U.R.C.) is formally constituted, organized and approved by the hospital's medical staff and governing body with the responsibility for the mechanisms needed to assure proper utilization of hospital services.

2. Documentation that the U.R.C. includes (or plans to include) broad specialty representation of the medical staff.

3. Documentation that the U.R. program insures (or has the capability to insure) that decisions on medical questions are made solely by the medical staff members.

4. Documentation that the U.R.C. meets customarily, at least monthly, with regular attendance of members.

5. Documentation that physicians do not have a vote in decisions concerning review of their own cases.

6. Assurance that the U.R.C. and the U.R. program receives administrative support deemed necessary by the medical staff.

7. Documentation that the hospital employes a U.R. Coordinator or identifies an employee who has responsibility for daily review coordination and communication with the Review Organization.

- 7 -

B. Procedural Criteria

1. Ability for correct usage of intensity of services and levels
    of care criteria. This includes the ability to reassess and
    modify length-of-stay certifications according to current
    information about an individual case.

2. Ability for correct usage of Review Organization forms.

3. Ability for correct usage of Review Organization's review
    procedures for timeliness of reviews, advance notification,
    appeal periods, extensions, and final notifications.

4. Ability to provide the Review Organization with accurate and
    timely statistical data on cases reviewed.

C. Measurement Criterion

1. Participating hospitals will be evaluated with the following
    Measurement Criterion to qualify for delegated status for
    concurrent review:

    Less than 2.5% disagreement rate for approved cases vs. non-
    approved cases between the Participating Hospital and the
    Review Organization.

2. Participating Hospitals will be evaluated with the following
    Measurement Criterion to maintain delegated status for
    concurrent review:

    Less than 2.5% disagreement rate for approved vs. non-
    approved days of care between the Participating Hospital and
    the Review Organization.

VII. PARTICIPATING PROVIDER COMMITTEE

A. A committee composed equally of Participating Hospitals and
    Participating Physicians shall be appointed by the Blue Cross
    Board of Directors by January 1, 1984. The Committee shall be
    known as the Prudent Buyer Plan Participating Provider Committee
    (Committee) and shall advise the Blue Cross Board of Directors
    and Blue Cross staff on Utilization Review policies, procedures
    and screening criteria as established and administered pursuant
    to this Exhibit C, Exhibit D, and Article VII.

B. Until such time as the Committee is appointed, the Blue Cross of
    California Physician Advisory Committee and Hospital Relations
    Committee shall act in the Committee's place.

C. The Committee shall consist of twenty-six (26) Members. Twelve
(12) participating physicians shall be appointed: One (1) each
from among Participating Physicians nominated by the County
Medical Societies in each of the Council Districts of the
California Medical Association, with one (1) Participating
Physician appointed from each California Medical Association
Council District, and one additional physician shall be
appointed from among Participating Physicians nominated by the
medical staff organizations of Participating teaching
hospitals.

Twelve (12) representatives of Participating Hospitals shall be
appointed. Four each shall be from among those nominated by the
Hospital Council of Northern California and the Hospital Council
of Southern California and two each shall be from among those
nominated by the Hospital Council of Central California and the
Hospital Council of San Diego and Imperial Counties.

The Chairman and Vice Chairman of the Committee, one of whom
shall be a Participating Physician and one of whom shall be a
representative of a Participating Hospital, shall be appointed
by the Blue Cross Board of Directors from among hospital
representatives and physicians who are members of at least one
of the following:

> The Blue Cross of California Board of Directors, the
> Blue Cross of Northern California Board of Directors,
> the Blue Cross of Southern California Board of Directors,
> the Blue Cross of California Physician Advisory Committee,
> or the Blue Cross of California Hospital Relations
> Committee.

Appointments shall be for three year terms, with initial
appointments staggered for one, two and three year appointments.

EXHIBIT D

DIAGNOSIS AND PROCEDURES
REQUIRING PREADMISSION REVIEW

The diagnosis and procedures listed below should receive preadmission review and authorization for guaranteed payment on inpatient hospitalization. They are divided into the following three categories:

Category I: Medical Necessity

   Procedures always requiring prior authorization for the medical necessity of inpatient care.

Category II: Procedures Customarily Performed in an Ambulatory Setting

   Procedures generally performed in an ambulatory setting which require prior authorization, based upon documentation of extra risk factors, for guaranteed payment of inpatient care.

Category III: May be Excluded as Inpatient Benefit in the Benefit Agreement

   Diagnosis and procedures which may be excluded as contract benefits for inpatient care in the Blue Cross Benefit Agreement.

CATEGORY I: MEDICAL NECESSITY

1. Scheduled procedure or treatment requiring hospitalization but not due to be performed within twenty-four (24) hours of admission

2. Non-emergency psychiatric admissions

3. Bunionectomy

4. Frenulectomy

5. Gynecomastia excision

6. Hammertoe repair with tenotomies and resection of bone

7. Submucous resection of nasal septum

8. Chemical dependency admissions

- 1 -

CATEGORY II: PROCEDURES CUSTOMARILY PERFORMED IN AN AMBULATORY SETTING

1. Integumentary System

   Breast biopsy - incision, excision (uni or bilateral)
   Excision of sebaceous cyst
   Mandible cyst excision - simple
   Pilonidal cyst excision, simple
   Simple excision, lymph node
   Skin graft, small
   Treatment of condylomata acuminate (male/female)

2. Musculoskeletal System

   Arthrodesis, fingers or toes
   Arthroplasty, small joints
   Arthroscopy of the knee where definitive procedure not planned
   Arthrotomy, small joint
   Bone marrow biopsy
   Bursectomy (simple)
   Capsulectomy/Capsulotomy, small joints
   Chondroplasty by arthroscopy
   Chronic pain evaluation plus rehabilitation
   Foreign body removal, superficial
   Fusion of small joints (i.e., interphalangeal)
   Ganglionectomy
   Joint manipulation
   Muscle biopsy
   Neuroma excision (Mortons and cutaneous and digital nerves)
   Ostectomy metatarsal (metatarsal head excision)
   Osteotomy
   Phalangectomy, partial or total
   Scar revision
   Simple exostosectomy of small bones
   Surgical aftercare, superficial wire removal, extremity
   Synovectomy - simple
   Tendon sheath release (De Quervains)
   Tenotomy hands, fingers, ankles, feet and toes
   Trigger finger release
   Zygoma (Zygomatic arch) reduction (simple)

3. Respiratory System

   Bronchoscopy
   Laryngoscopy as an only procedure

4. Cardiovascular System

   Routine cardiovascular non-invasive diagnostic procedures
   Temporal artery, ligation or biopsy
   Varicose vein ligation

- 2 -

5. Digestive System

   Branchial arch appendage excision (simple)
   Colostomy revision (simple)
   Fistulectomy (small)
   Gastrointestinal endoscopy (uncomplicated)
   Liver biopsy, percutaneous
   Paracentesis
   Rectal polypectomy (simple)
   Sigmoidoscopy
   Wedge resection of lip

6. Urinary System

   Cystoscopy
   Meatotomy
   Urethral dilatation

7. Male Genital System

   Circumcision
   Hydrocele excision
   Prostate biopsy, needle
   Vasectomy

8. Female Genital System

   Abortion, Therapeutic (1st trimester)
   Biopsy of cervix, endometrium, (endometrial aspiration or washing), vagina
   Cauterization of cervix
   Circumferential conization
   Cryotherapy with biopsy and/or endocervical curettage
   Culdoscopy (culdocentesis)
   Dilatation and curettage (diagnositc or therapeutic)
   Fulguration, vulva and cervix
   Hymenotomy
   Hysterosalpinogram
   Laparoscopy
   Pelvic exam under anesthesia
   Removal of IUD
   Tubal ligation
   Use of laser in treating lesions of cervix, vagina or vulva
   Vaginal stenosis release (simple)
   Vaginal-tumor (cyst) excision
   Vulva (labial) biopsy

9. Nervous System

   Decompression of the Medial Nerve at the Carpal Tunnel
   Nerve biopsy
   Nerve block
   Nerve repair, simple
   Neurectomy
   Neurolysis, simple

- 3 -

10. Eye and Ocular Adnexa System

    Cataract excision by phako-emulsification with/without implant
    Chalazion excision
    Discission lens (needling of lens)
    Ectropion/entropion repair
    Foreign body removal
    Lacrimal duct probing
    Pterygium (excision or transposition)
    Tarsorrhaphy

11. Otorhinolaryngology (Ear, Nose, Throat)

    Antral puncture
    Resection of turbinate
    Inferior turbinate fracture
    Myringoplasty
    Nasal polypectomy (small or few)
    Nose, closed reduction
    Otoscopy, with or without removal of foreign body
    Tongue biopsy

CATEGORY III: MAY BE EXCLUDED AS INPATIENT BENEFIT

The following diagnosis and procedures are generally excluded from Blue Cross
Benefit Agreements:

1. Allergy and environmental control

2. Behavior problems

3. Blepharoplasty (upper, lower or combined)

4. Chelation therapy for other than acute metal toxicity (e.g., ASHD)

5. Cosmetic or reconstructive surgery -- all types

6. Developmental problem(s)

7. Eating disorder(s)

8. Facial dermabrasion

9. Learning disability(ies)

10. Mammoplasty (augmentation)

11. Obesity

12. Otoplasty (unilateral/bilateral)

13. Rhytidectomy

14. Vermilionectomy

Blue Cross of California

EXHIBIT E

ARBITRATION FOR UTILIZATION REVIEW

The initial decision regarding whether Hospital Services or Medical Services are Medically Necessary shall be made pursuant to Section 7.2. PHYSICIAN may appeal such a decision pursuant to the terms of Section 7.5. Arbitration under that section shall follow the procedures below:

A. PHYSICIAN, agrees to submit any dispute concerning a Utilization Review decision, unresolved by reconsideration or review pursuant to the terms of Section 7.2, to binding arbitration. The arbitration shall be commenced by PHYSICIAN making written demand on BLUE CROSS. The scope of that arbitration shall be limited to a determination of whether, or to what extent, benefits specified in the applicable Prudent Buyer Benefit Agreement were Medically Necessary or otherwise payable for the claim or claims in dispute.

B. The arbitration shall be held before a neutral arbitrator appointed by the county medical association of the county in which the services were provided. If the county medical association declines or is unble to appoint an arbitrator, the arbitrator shall be appointed by the superior court having jurisdiction over the matter according to California Code of Civil Procedure Section 1281.6, or as otherwise mutually agreed in writing by BLUE CROSS and PHYSICIAN.

C. Any arbitration shall be conducted according to the California Arbitration Act, Code of Civil Procedure Section 1280 et seq., or as otherwise mutually agreed. PHYSICIAN and BLUE CROSS agree that the arbitration findings shall be binding upon any subsequent litigation.

APPENDIX D

Universal Health Network, Inc., Hospital Agreement

Universal Health Network, Inc. Hospital Agreement

UNIVERSAL HEALTH NETWORK, INC., hereinafter referred to as "UHN," and _____ , hereinafter referred to as "Hospital," agree as follows:

Recital of Facts

WHEREAS, UHN is a California non-profit corporation comprised of licensed acute care general hospitals and provider physician, dentist and podiatrist members whose purpose is to support the provision of health care services by its members by means of agreements with health care insurers and self-insured employee benefit health care plans, hereinafter called "insurers and plans."

WHEREAS, Hospital is a duly licensed acute care hospital member of UHN.

WHEREAS, Hospital wishes to contract with UHN so that Hospital may provide its services to insurers and plans and accept as payment in full for such services the amounts set forth in this Agreement.

WHEREAS, UHN wishes to contract with Hospital so that UHN may effectively support the provision of Hospital's services to insurers and plans.

THEREFORE, in consideration for the mutual covenants and agreements contained herein, it is hereby agreed as follows:

1. *SERVICES.*

    a. UHN agrees to include Hospital in its list of hospitals from which insurers and plans select hospital providers and shall continue to seek out and contract with insurers and providers which utilize such list. Hospital understands that it may be removed from such list upon its breach of the terms and conditions of this Agreement, or upon suspension or termination of its membership in UHN.

b. Hospital agrees to provide its usual and customary hospital services, consistent with standards set by the Joint Commission on Accreditation of Hospitals and the laws of the State of California, to subscribers of insurers and plans hereinafter called "Subscribers," which have contracted with UHN for the services of UHN members, provided that Hospital may refuse to provide such services under any UHN contract if Hospital provides written notice of such refusal to UHN within ten (10) days of notification from UHN of any UHN contract. Hospital hereby authorizes UHN to represent Hospital in regards to the negotiation and entry into such contracts with insurers and plans.

c. Hospital understands that UHN encourages its providers to provide services under this Agreement in the most cost efficient and economical manner. To that end, Hospital shall provide the services set forth in Paragraph 1.b of this Agreement at rates or discounts comparable or lower than rates or discounts it offers to or accepts from any other hospital based preferred provider organization. For the purposes of this Agreement, "hospital based preferred provider organization" shall mean any preferred provider organization which is controlled by or whose expenses are provided in most part by licensed hospitals.

2. *ELIGIBILITY.* Hospital agrees to accept determination of insurers and plans of subscriber eligibility and agrees to verify such eligibility upon admission.

3. *COMPENSATION.* Hospital agrees to compensate directly to Pacific Health Resources, 1423 South Grand Avenue, Los Angeles, California 90015, the amount of twenty-five hundred dollars ($2,500.00) per month for management and administration services to UHN. PHR shall bill Hospital not later than the fifteenth (15th) of the month for the cost of services for the preceding

month. Hospital shall make payments on such billing within fifteen (15) days of receipt.

4. *PAYMENT TO HOSPITAL BY INSURERS AND PLANS.* Hospital agrees to accept as payment in full for its services the amounts set forth in the UHN Provider Agreement with the insurers and plans. It is understood that insurers shall require assignment by its subscribers to Hospital of subscribers right to indemnification for all services rendered under the coverage amount. Hospital shall make no claims against subscribers for services rendered for which payment has been received. It is understood that UHN is in no way responsible for payment by insurers and plans for services rendered by Hospital.

It is understood that in accordance with terms of the insurance policy or health plan, on or before thirty (30) days following receipt of a claim form from Hospital, insurers and plans agree to make payment to Hospital for hospital services provided to subscribers for the services for which coverage is verified. Hospital agrees to make every reasonable effort to submit all claims to insurers and plans no later than sixty (60) days from the date of service given to the subscriber.

5. *UTILIZATION REVIEW.* Hospital agrees to participate in and cooperate with utilization review programs established by UHN.

6. *THIRD PARTY BENEFITS.*

a. If any benefits to which insurer and plan subscribers are entitled under this Agreement are also covered under any other health benefit plan, or insurance policy, or subject to third party liability, insurers and plans, UHN and Hospital shall make best efforts to reduce benefits hereunder to the extent that benefits or claim are available to subscribers under such other plan, policy or liability whether or not a claim is made for the same.

b. In the event of third party liability, Worker's Compensation claims, or other primary insurance coverage, Hospital shall make no demand upon insurers or plans for reimbursement until all primary sources of payment have been pursued and it is determined that full payment cannot be obtained. In the cases in which Hospital demands reimbursement from insurer or plan, Hospital shall subrogate its claim to insurer or plan and Hospital shall assist and continue to assist insurer or plan in its collection efforts by providing appropriate bills, invoices and documents as are available.

c. None of the above rules as to coordination of benefits will serve as a barrier to the subscriber first receiving direct health services which are covered in this Agreement.

7. *TERM.* The term of this Agreement shall be for a period of time of one (1) year commencing on _____, and shall automatically renew on a year to year basis unless written notice of termination is provided pursuant to Paragraph 8 of this Agreement.

8. *TERMINATION.* Either party may terminate this Agreement upon sixty (60) days notice to the other party with or without cause.

9. *HOSPITAL-PATIENT RELATIONSHIP.* It is understood that Hospital shall maintain a hospital-patient relationship with subscribers and shall be solely responsible to the subscribers for hospital services and treatment. It is expressly agreed that Hospital is an independent contractor and that insurers and plans and UHN shall have no dominion or control over Hospital, the hospital-patient relationship, the Hospital's personnel or facilities. It is further understood that insurers and plans nor their third party administrators are associated, employed or acting as a representative for Hospital and do not exercise any control or direction over Hospital or the services Hospital renders.

10. *AMENDMENT.* This agreement may be amended only upon the mutual written consent of the parties.

11. *INDEPENDENT CONTRACTOR.* No relationship of em-

ployer or employee is created by this Agreement, it being understood that UHN and its employees and agents will act hereunder as independent contractors, and shall not have any claim under this Agreement or otherwise against Hospital for vacation pay, sick leave, retirement benefits, Social Security, Worker's Compensation benefits or employee benefits of any kind. During the term of this Agreement, or any renewals hereof, UHN shall be fully responsible and liable for any and all State and Federal income or other taxes to which payments made hereunder by Hospital to UHN may become subject.

12. *INDEMNITY.* Hospital shall hold harmless and indemnify UHN from any claims, losses, damages, liabilities, costs, expenses or obligations arising out of or resulting from the provision of health care services by Hospital to the subscribers of insurers and plans. Hospital shall carry professional and general comprehensive liability insurance in amounts satisfactory to UHN.

13. *NOTICE.* Any notice, request, demand or other communication required or permitted hereunder shall be deemed to be properly given when delivered personally or on the next business day after it is deposited in the United States mail, postage prepaid, to the address of UHN or Hospital stated in this Agreement, or such other address as may hereafter be specified by notice in writing.

14. *ARBITRATION.* The parties hereto agree to arbitration of contract disputes. Disputes between Hospital and UHN arising out of or resulting from the provisions of this contract will be determined by submission to arbitration and not by a lawsuit or resort to court process except as California law provides for judicial review of arbitration proceedings. Within fifteen (15) days after any of the above named parties shall give notice to the other of demand for arbitration of said controversy, the parties to the controversy shall each appoint an arbitrator and give notice of such appointment to the other. Within a reasonable time after such notices have been given, the two (2) arbitrators so selected shall select a neutral arbitrator and give notice of selection thereof to the

parties. The arbitrators shall hold a hearing within a reasonable time from the date of notice of selection of the neutral arbitrator. All notices shall be served by United States mail. The arbitration shall be compulsory and binding and, except as provided herein, shall be conducted and governed by California law. Hospital and UHN are hereby giving up their constitutional right to have any such dispute decided in a court of law before a jury and instead are accepting use of arbitration.

15. *ENTIRE AGREEMENT.* This Agreement supersedes any and all other Agreements, either oral or in writing, between the parties hereto and contains all of the covenants and agreements between them. Each party acknowledges that no representation, inducement, promise or agreement, orally or otherwise, has been made by any party, or anyone acting on behalf of any party, which is not embodied herein. Any modification of this Agreement will be effective only if it is in writing and signed by the party to be charged.

16. *SEVERABILITY.* If any provision in this Agreement is held to be invalid, void, or unenforceable, the remaining provisions shall nevertheless continue in full force and effect without being impaired or invalidated in any way.

17. *GOVERNING LAW.* This Agreement is entered into and shall be governed by and construed in accordance with the laws of the State of California.

18. *MEDICARE DISCLOSURE PROVISIONS.*

a. UHN agrees, in connection with the subject matter of this Agreement, to cooperate fully with Hospital by, among other things, maintaining and making available all necessary records, in order to assure that Hospital will be able to meet all requirements for participation and payment associated with public or private third party payment programs including, but not limited to, matters covered by Section 1861( ) (1) (I) of the Social Security Act.

b. For the purpose of implementing Section 1861(v)(1)(I) of the Social Security Act, as amended, and any written regulations thereto, UHN agrees to comply with the following statutory requirements governing the maintenance of documentation to verify the cost of services rendered under this Agreement:

"(i) until the expiration of four years after the furnishing of such services pursuant to such contract, UHN shall make available, upon written request to the Secretary or upon request to the Comptroller General, or any of their duly authorized representatives, the contracts, books, documents and records of UHN that are necessary to certify the nature and extent of such costs, and

(ii) if UHN carries out any of the duties of the contract through a subcontract with a value or cost of $10,000 or more over a twelve month period, with a related organization [as that term is defined with regard to a provider in 42 C.F.R. §405.427(b)], such subcontract shall contain a clause to the effect that until the expiration of four years after the furnishing of such services pursuant to such subcontract, the related organization shall make available, upon written request to the Secretary, or upon request to the Comptroller General, or any of their duly authorized representatives, the subcontract, and books, documents and records of such organization that are necessary to verify the nature and extent of such costs."

c. If UHN is requested to disclose books, documents or records pursuant to this provision for purpose of an audit, UHN shall notify Hospital of the nature and scope of such request and UHN shall make available, upon written request of Hospital, all such books, documents or records, during regular business hours of UHN.

d. In the event of any breach of this Paragraph by UHN, or any subcontractor of UHN, Hospital shall have the right to terminate this Agreement after ten (10) days' notice to UHN.

e. UHN shall indemnify and hold harmless Hospital in the event that any amount of reimbursement is denied or disallowed because of the failure of UHN or any subcontractor of UHN to comply with its obligations to maintain and make available books, documents or records pursuant to this provision. Such indemnity shall include, but not be limited to, the amount of reimbursement denied, plus any interest, penalties, and reasonable attorneys' fees.

f. This provision pertains solely to the maintenance and disclosure of specified records and shall have no effect on the right of the parties to this Agreement to make assignments or delegations.

IN WITNESS WHEREOF, the parties hereto have executed this Agreement on the _____ day of _____ , 19 _____ .

UNIVERSAL HEALTH NETWORK, INC.

By _____

Address:

1423 South Grand Avenue
Los Angeles, California 90015

HOSPITAL

By _____

Address:

Universal Health Network, Inc.
Hospital Provider Membership Application

This is an application for a hospital provider membership in Universal Health Network.

As a member, this Hospital agrees to abide by the Articles of Incorporation, Bylaws, and any Rules and Regulations of Universal Health Network. Copies of these documents have been made available to this Hospital for review. This Hospital further agrees to abide by the provisions of the Universal Health Network, Inc. Hospital Agreement which has been signed by this Hospital. This Hospital agrees to participate in and cooperate with Utilization Review Programs established by UHN.

This Hospital understands and agrees that any disputes arising out of this application for membership, or membership in Universal Health Network shall be resolved by the grievance and arbitration procedures, as provided in the Universal Health Network Bylaws.

NAME OF HOSPITAL:

ADDRESS:

TELEPHONE:

DATE: ─────────────────────────────────────

BY: ──

TITLE: ───────────────────────────────────────

SPONSOR'S SIGNATURE ───────────────────────

UHN PRESIDENT'S SIGNATURE ──────────────────

APPENDIX E

Directory of PPOs*

*The information in this section appears with the cooperation and permission of the Clearinghouse on PPOs of the Institute for International Health Initiatives, Inc., an affiliate of the American Medical Care and Review Association (AMCRA). We thank that organization for its help in making this available.

ALABAMA

Dynamic Health Services, Ltd.
3010 Stockton Hill Road
Suite D
Kingman, Arizona 86401
(602) 753-3636
Contact Person:
M. Azam Khan, M.D.
Medical Director
Status:
Operational
Nature of Sponsorship:
Clinic/Emergency Medical Facility

ARIZONA

Physicians Quality Care Group, Inc.
101-A Lowe Avenue
Huntsville, Alabama 35801
(205) 539-3851
Contact Person:
Lary Sullivan, M.D.
Status:
Operational
Nature of Sponsorship:
Physician

Southern Arizona Physicians' Service
Association
400 E. Broadway, Suite 308
Tucson, Arizona 85711
(602) 326-0455
Contact Person:
Thomas P. Finley
Executive Director
Status:
Pre-Operational
Nature of Sponsorship:
Blue Cross/Blue Shield

Valley Independent Physicians
5025 E. Washington Street #112
Phoenix, Arizona 85034
(602) 244-0233
Contact Person:
Frederic L. Snowden
Status:
Pre-Operational
Nature of Sponsorship:
Physician

CALIFORNIA

Benefit Panel Services
1000 West Ninth Street
Los Angeles, California 90015
(213) 627-3415
Contact Person:
Terry L. Worthylake
Executive Vice President
Status:
Operational
Nature of Sponsorship:
Physician

Blue Cross of California
1950 Franklin Street
Oakland, California 94659
(415) 645-3603
Contact Person:
Leona M. Butler
Dir. Provider Contracting
Status:
Pre-Operational
Nature of Sponsorship:
Hospital Service Plan

California Health Network
630 Leavenworth Street
Suite 1

San Francisco, California 94109
(415) 474-1246
Contact Person:
Philip M. Levine
Status:
Operational
Nature of Sponsorship:
Hospital

California Preferred Professionals, Inc.
415 West Carroll Avenue
Suite 102
Glendora, California 91740
(213) 914-4871
Contact Person:
Edward Zalta, M.D., President
Paul S. Parry, Exec. Dir.
Status:
Operational
Nature of Sponsorship:
Physician

CarePlus
20500 Nordhoff
Chatsworth, California 91311
(213) 700-2105
Contact Person:
Layton Crouch
Status:
Pre-Operational
Nature of Sponsorship:
Hospitals/ Health Care Related
  Ventures

Charter Medical Preferred Provider
  Organization
21520 S. Pioneer Boulevard
Suite 307
Hawaiian Gardens, California 90716
(213) 865-0832

Contact Person:
Paul S. Bodner
Executive Director
Status:
Operational
Nature of Sponsorship:
Charter Medical Corporation

Community Referral Service
310 Tahiti Way, Suite 316
Marina del Rey, California 90291
(213) 306-1872
Contact Person:
William G. West, Ph.D.
Executive Director
Status:
Operational
Nature of Sponsorship:
American Board of Psychotherapy

Diablo Valley PPO
P.O. Box 1028
Martinez, California 94553
(415) 372-8381
Contact Person:
Carole Stewart
Status:
Pre-Operational
Nature of Sponsorship:
Physician/ Diablo Valley IPA

Greater San Diego Preferred Provider
  Organization
3702 Ruffin Road
San Diego, California 92123
(619) 292-0301
Contact Person:
James G. Stumpfel or
Paul Ridgely
Status:

Pre-Operational
Nature of Sponsorship:
HMO/IPA

Integrative Healthcare Center
500 West Santa Ana Boulevard
Fourth Floor
Santa Ana, California 92701
(714) 973-9355
Contact Person:
Sandra Gordon
Executive Administrator
Status:
Pre-Operational
Nature of Sponsorship:
Physician

Lakewood Physicians Association
3650 E. South Street
Suite 301
Lakewood, California 90712
(213) 634-7333
Contact Person:
Ronald Fischman, M.D.
Chairman
Status:
Pre-Operational
Nature of Sponsorship:
Physician

Long Beach Memorial Medical Group,
    Inc.
P.O. Box 90576
Long Beach, California 90809-0576
(213) 595-3984
Contact Person:
Patraig Carney, M.D.
President
Status:
Pre-Operational
Nature of Sponsorship:
Physician Professional Corp.

Nature of Sponsorship:
Physician Professional Corp.

Med Network
1200 North Main
Suite 424
Santa Ana, California 92701
(714) 953-9600
Contact Person:
Richard Toral
Status:
Operational
Nature of Sponsorship:
Private Enterprise

Medical Care Foundation of
    Sacramento
5030 El Camino Avenue
Carmichael, California 95608
(916) 971-9231
Contact Person:
Ms. Diane Rice
Status:
Pre-Operational
Nature of Sponsorship:
FMC

Mid-Coast PPO
P.O. Box 308
Salinas, California 93902
(408) 455-1833
Contact Person:
Ed Colvin
Status:
Pre-Operational
Nature of Sponsorship:
Physician

P.P.O., Inc.
1390 Market Street

Suite 911
San Francisco, California 94102
(415) 864-5501
Contact Person:
Rodrick J. Hinshaw, M.D., President
John L. Chapman, Dir. Mkg.
Status:
Operational
Nature of Sponsorship:
United Foundations for Medical Care

San Diego PPO, Inc.
P.O. Box 23015
San Diego, California 92123
(619) 565-9255
Contact Person:
Gus Anderson
Lowell Foster
Status:
Operational
Nature of Sponsorship:
San Diego FMC

Select Health
2485 Clay Street
San Francisco, California 94115
(415) 563-4321
Contact Person:
Pamela Berven
Executive Director
Status:
Operational
Nature of Sponsorship:
Physician/Hospital

SelectCare
7840 Firestone Boulevard
Downey, California 90241
(213) 861-5353
Contact Person:

John Miller
Status:
Pre-Operational
Nature of Sponsorship:
Medical Group

Sonoma Foundation Preferred
 Provider Organization
3033 Cleveland Avenue
Santa Rosa, California 95401
(707) 544-2010
Contact Person:
Gene Scott
Executive Vice President
Status:
Operational
Nature of Sponsorship:
Physician

Universal Health Network
1423 South Grand Avenue
Los Angeles, California 90015
(213) 742-6245
Contact Person:
Nicholas Moss
Vice President
Status:
Pre-Operational
Nature of Sponsorship:
Physician/Hospital

COLORADO

Araphoe IPA
777 E. Gerard Avenue
Englewood, Colorado 80110
(303) 789-6322
Contact Person:
Pete Baker, M.D.
President

Status:
Pre-Operational
Nature of Sponsorship:
Physician

Cherry Creek Associated Physicians,
Inc.
(Rose Medical Center PPO)
4567 East 9th Avenue
Denver, Colorado 80220
(303) 320-2031
Contact Person:
Nancy McCarroll
Manager
Status:
Operational
Nature of Sponsorship:
Hospital

Mountain Medical Affiliates, Inc.
1850 Williams Street
Denver, Colorado 80218
(303) 831-7327
Contact Person:
Tobie Miller
Status:
Operational
Nature of Sponsorship:
Physician/Hospital

Preferred Healthcare, Inc.
2310 North Tejon Street
Colorado Springs, Colorado 80907
(303) 630-5469
Contact Person:
Pat Steele
Status:
Operational
Nature of Sponsorship:
Physician

DISTRICT OF COLUMBIA
PriMed Health Plan
1101 Thirtieth Street, NW
Suite 108
Washington, DC 20007
(202) 333-9300
Contact Person:
Dennis Fauk
Status:
Pre-Operational
Nature of Sponsorship:
Physician

FLORIDA

AV Medical Health Plan
9400 South Dadeland Boulevard
Miami, Florida 33156
(305) 665-5437
Contact Person:
Harvey Felser or
Robert Jones
Status:
Operational
Nature of Sponsorship:
HMO

Blue Cross and Blue Shield of Florida
P.O. Box 1798
Jacksonville, Florida 32231
(904) 791-6485
Contact Person:
V. Paul Mitalas
Director of PPO Analysis
Status:
Pre-Operational
Nature of Sponsorship:
Health Insurance Plan

Health Providers, Inc.
1400 Northwest 12th Avenue
Miami, Florida 33136
(305) 325-5296
Contact Person:
Carol Gleber
Administrator
Status:
Operational
Nature of Sponsorship:
Physician/Hospital

Individual Option Plan
P.O. Box 2268
Pompano Beach, Florida 33061
(305) 943-0102
Contact Person:
Stu Johnson
Status:
Operational
Nature of Sponsorship:
Humana, Inc.

Southeastern Medical Center
(No official name yet)
1750 NE 167th Street
North Miami Beach, Florida 33162
(305) 945-5400
Contact Person:
Rebecca Burke
Dir., Develop. & Mktg.
Status:
Pre-Operational
Nature of Sponsorship:
Hospital

GEORGIA

Greater Atlanta Physicians Association
805 Peachtree Street

Atlanta, Georgia 30308
(404) 881-8196
Contact Person:
George Swerdloff
Status:
Pre-Operational
Nature of Sponsorship:
Physician

Medical Cost Management Systems, Inc.
1147-A Henry Avenue
Columbus, Georgia 31906
(404) 323-6154
Contact Person:
William Amos, Jr., M.D.
Medical Director
Status:
Operational
Nature of Sponsorship:
Third Party Administrator

Psychiatric Providers of Georgia
Northcreek Bldg. 100, Ste. 102
3715 Northside Pkwy.
Atlanta, Georgia 30327
(404) 261-2880
Contact Person:
Charles H. Hendry, M.D.
Medical Director
Status:
Operational
Nature of Sponsorship:
IPA

ILLINOIS

Christie Clinic Association
104 West Clark Street
Champaign, Illinois 61820

(217) 351-1200
Contact Person:
Robert P. Thompson
Status:
Operational
Nature of Sponsorship:
Multi-Specialty Medical Group

Northside Preferred Provider
   Organization
4640 North Marine Drive
Chicago, Illinois 60640
(312) 728-7877
Contact Person:
Gerald M. Berkowitz, M.D.
Status:
Operational
Nature of Sponsorship:
Physician Primary Care

INDIANA

Mirich Medical Corporation
521 East 86th Avenue
Suite E
Merrillville, Indiana 46410
(219) 769-3553
Contact Person:
Eleanor Kay-Mirich
Health Administrator
Status:
Pre-Operational
Nature of Sponsorship:
Physician

KENTUCKY

Physicians Alliance for Medical
   Excellence, Inc.
1725 Harrodsburg Road

Suite 202
Lexington, Kentucky 40504
(606) 276-2203
Contact Person:
John Hackworth, Ph.D.
Executive Director
Status:
Operational
Nature of Sponsorship:
Physician

LOUISIANA

Ochsner Clinic PPO
1514 Jefferson Highway
New Orleans, Louisiana 70121
(504) 838-4000
Contact Person:
Jim Winfield
PPO Manager
Status:
Operational
Nature of Sponsorship:
Physician

Oschner Foundation Hospital PPO
1516 Jefferson Highway
New Orleans, Louisiana 70121
(504) 838-3000
Contact Person:
Jim Winfield
Status:
Operational
Nature of Sponsorship:
Physician

MARYLAND

American Health Network, Inc.
6201 Greenbelt Road

U-8A
College Park, Maryland 20740
(301) 474-4600
Contact Person:
Ann A. Hodgkinson
Status:
Pre-Operational
Nature of Sponsorship:
Physician/Other Health Professionals

Preferred Care, Inc.
6611 Kenilworth Avenue
Suite 400
Riverdale, Maryland 20737
(301) 277-6520
Contact Person:
Robert Helfrich
Status:
Pre-Operational
Nature of Sponsorship:
Physician

MASSACHUSETTS

John Hancock
P.O. Box 111
Boston, Massachusetts 02117
(617) 421-4700
Contact Person:
John K. Cross
Status:
Pre-Operational
Nature of Sponsorship:
Insurance Carrier

MINNESOTA

Minnesota Health Network, Inc.
2221 University Avenue, SE
Suite 123

Minneapolis, Minnesota 55414
(612) 623-3400
Contact Person:
Gary F. Gray
Status:
Pre-Operational
Nature of Sponsorship:
Physician

Select Care PPO
800 East 28th Street at Chicago Avenue
Minneapolis, Minnesota 55407
(612) 874-5107
Contact Person:
Helen Yates
Executive Director
Status:
Pre-Operational
Nature of Sponsorship:
Hospital/Physician

MISSISSIPPI

Individual Option Plan
1037 North Flowood Drive
Jackson, Mississippi 39208
(601) 932-5400
Contact Person:
Joe Sharp
Status:
Operational
Nature of Sponsorship:
Humana, Inc.

MISSOURI

Preferred Health Professionals
6601 Rockhill Road
Kansas City, Missouri 64131
(816) 361-0133

Contact Person:
Kathleen O'Connor
Executive Director
Status:
Operational
Nature of Sponsorship:
Physician/Hospital

NEW JERSEY

New Jersey Blue Shield
33 Washington
Newark, New Jersey 07102
(201) 456-2568
Contact Person:
G.E. Grashorn
Status:
Pre-Operational
Nature of Sponsorship:
Blue Shield/Physician

NEW YORK

Four Winds Hospital
Katonah, New York 10536
(914) 763-8151
Contact Person:
Diane Biumi, Medical Records
Michael C. Piercey, M.D.
Status:
Pre-Operational
Nature of Sponsorship:
Hospital

OHIO

Coalition for Cost Effective Health
Services
285 East Main
Columbus, Ohio 43215

(614) 221-1381
Contact Person:
Charles A. Turner, III
Executive Director
Status:
Pre-Operational
Nature of Sponsorship:
Community Based

Hillcrest Preferred Provider
Organization
6780 Mayfield Road
Mayfield Heights, Ohio 44124
(216) 449-4500
Contact Person:
Paul R. Zeit, M.D.
Status:
Operational
Nature of Sponsorship:
Physician/Hospital

Medical Mutual of Cleveland, Inc.
2060 East Ninth Street
Cleveland, Ohio 44115
(216) 687-6857
Contact Person:
Roger Cooley
Status:
Pre-Operational
Nature of Sponsorship:
Blue Cross/Blue Shield

Northern Ohio Health Providers
Organization, Inc.
Marymount Hospital
12300 McCracken Road
Garfield Heights, Ohio 44125
(216) 662-2059
Contact Person:
Dale H. Cowan, M.D., J.D.
President

Status:
Operational
Nature of Sponsorship:
Physician

Ohio Health Choice Plan
2351 East 22nd Street
Cleveland, Ohio 44115
(216) 781-6427
Contact Person:
Robert P. Page
Status:
Operational
Nature of Sponsorship:
Hospital

Tri-Med Affiliates, Inc.
11201 Shaker Boulevard
Cleveland, Ohio 44104
(216) 368-7318
Contact Person:
Philip A. Newbold
Status:
Pre-Operational
Nature of Sponsorship:
Hospital

Western Reserve Health Provider
Organization, Inc. & St.
Joseph Riverside Hospital PPO
1300 Tod Avenue, NW
Warren, Ohio 44485
(216) 394-6565
Contact Person:
Joseph Colosi
Administrative Director
Status:
Operational
Nature of Sponsorship:
Physician/ Hosp. Participation

OKLAHOMA

Comprehensive Medical Care Affiliates,
Inc. (CompMed, Inc.)
P.O. Box 14044
Tulsa, Oklahoma 74159
(918) 587-0272
Contact Person:
Donald A. Penn, President
Wes Conley, Executive VP
Status:
Operational
Nature of Sponsorship:
Hospital

PPO of Tulsa
1120 South Utica Avenue
Tulsa, Oklahoma 74104
(918) 584-1351
Contact Person:
Scott P. Serota
Status:
Pre-Operational
Nature of Sponsorship:
Hospital/Physician

PENNSYLVANIA

Pennsylvania Preferred Professionals
1211 Lakemont Road
Villa Nova, Pennsylvania 19085
(215) 527-0222
Contact Person:
Joseph Nowaslawski, M.D.
Status:
Pre-Operational
Nature of Sponsorship:
Physician

VIRGINIA

KeyCare
2015 Staples Mill Road
P.O. Box 27401
Richmond, Virginia 23279
(804) 359-7488
Contact Person:
James L. Gore
Vice President
Status:
Pre-Operational
Nature of Sponsorship:
Blue Cross/Blue Shield

Bibliography

1. Aim PPOs At Business, Not Providers. *Modern Healthcare*. April 1983.
2. Anderson, A. R. Nonprofits: Check Your Attention to Customers. *Harvard Business Review*. May-June 1982.
3. Berger, Judith D. Selective Contracting: California's Hot Potato? *Hospital Forum*. November-December 1982.
4. Carroll, Marjorie Smith and Arnett, Ross H. III. Private Health Insurance Plans in 1978 and 1979: A Review of Coverage, Enrollment, and Financial Experience. *Health Care Financing Review*. September 1981.
5. Cassidy, Robert. Will the PPO Movement Freeze You Out? *Medical Economics*. April 18, 1983.
6. Coalitions Hungry for Hospital Data. *Modern Healthcare*. January 1983.
7. A Confidential Survey of Benefit Managers by Segal Associates. Martin E. Segal Company. August 1982.
8. Cunningham, Robert M., Jr. Changing Philosophies in Medical Care and the Rule of the Investor-Owned Hospital. *New England Journal of Medicine*. September 23, 1983.
9. Defining Our Own Future: An American Hospital Association Glossary. American Hospital Association. January 1983.

10. Denver PPOs Save One-Fifth On Bills. *Health Services Information*. July 5, 1982.
11. Doctors Hope Cut-Rate "Preferred Provider" Organizations Can Fill Empty Waiting Rooms. *Medical World News*. February 28, 1983.
12. Ellwein, Linda. Interstudy Internal Memo. February 1981.
13. Ellwein, Linda. Preferred Provider Organizations: A New Form of Competitive Health Plan? *Colorado Medicine*. March 1982.
14. Ellwood, Paul M., M.D. New Organizational Arrangements to Help Doctors and Hospitals Cope with HMOs, PPOs, DRGs and Medi-Cal. Presentation to Alternative Healthcare, Delivery Systems and Medicare in the 1980's. Universal City, California. January 27, 1983.
15. Enders, R. J. The Preferred Provider Organization—Pro-Competitive Alternative or Anti-Trust Problem? *Hospital Forum*. November-December 1982.
16. Finney, Robert. Interview. August 9, 1983.
17. Fox, Peter. Preferred Provider Organizations: A Progress Report. Associated Hospital Systems Trustee, Educational Conference on Private Sector Initiatives to Control Health Costs. Carefree, Arizona. March 15, 1983.
18. Freedland, Mark S. and Schendler, Carol Ellen. National Health Expenditures: Short-Term Outlook and Long-Term Projections. *Health Care Financing Review*. Winter 1981.
19. Glueck, David L. Trends in Health Care Costs. *Pension World*. November 1982.
20. Hadley, Jack; Feder, Judith; and Mullner, Ross. "Care for the Poor and Hospitals" Financial Status: Results of a Survey of Hospitals in Large Cities." Draft Report, undated.
21. Hatfield, John; Kubal, Joseph D. Preferred Provider Organizations. *Urban Health*. January 1983.
22. Havighurst, Clark C. and Hackbarth, Glenn M. Private Cost Containment. *New England Journal of Medicine*. June 7, 1979.
23. Health Care Industry, Business, Show Increasing Interest in PPO Concept. *FAH Review*. July/August 1982.
24. Hunt, David. Preferred Provider Organizations. *Private Practice*. November 1982.

25. Inglehart, John K. Health Policy Report. *New England Journal of Medicine.* January 27, 1983.
26. Inter Study Researchers Trace Progress of PPOs, Provide Insights Into Future Growth. *FAH Review.* July/August 1982.
27. Investor-Owned Hospitals Study PPO Concept; Leaders of Industry Adopt "Wait and See" Policy. *FAH Review.* July/August 1982.
28. Johnson, Donald E. L. Price Competition Will be Legacy of California's Medi-Cal Czar. *Modern Healthcare.* September 1982.
29. Johnson, Donald E. L. If Hospitals and Physicians Don't Grab the PPO Market, Insurers Will. *Modern Healthcare.* March 1983.
30. Johnson, Donald E. L. Nonprofit Networks Link Resources to Grab Piece of National Markets. *Modern Healthcare.* October 1982.
31. Johnson, Richard L. Health Care 2000 A.D.: The Impact of Conglomerates. *Hospital Progress.* April 1981.
32. Kaiser, Leland R. Innovation in the Hospital. *Hospital Forum.* March-April 1982; Dennis Strum, *et al,* An R&D System that Works: Lutheran Hospital Society Shares its Step-By-Step Process in Building its High-Results Program. *Hospital Forum.* March-April 1982.
33. Keppel, Bruce. Multiple-Employer Trusts Cause Concern: New Insurance Chief Vows to Monitor Health Plans. *LA Times.* May 3, 1983.
34. Kemezys, K. P. Hospital Construction Moratoriums and Preferred Provider Organizations are emerging issues in various states. *Health Law Virgil.* March 4, 1983.
35. Kodner, Karen. Competition, Getting a Fix on PPOs. *Hospitals. J.A.H.A.*
36. Koehn, Hank. Networking. Luthern Hospital Society Conference on Networking. Phoenix, Arizona. February 20, 1983.
37. Kopp, Walter C. Selective Contracting: Preparing Hospitals and Physicians. Arthur Young and Co. San Francisco. 1983.
38. Kuntz, Esther Fritz. Hospital Forming PPOs to Fend off HMO Rivals. *Modern Healthcare.* February 1983.
39. Lefton, D. Competitive Market Spawning PPOs. *American Medical News.* 25:7–8. May 7, 1983.

40. Maloney, Sheila A. Preferred Provider Organizations: An Overview for State Regulations. *The New Times.* National Association of Health Maintenance Organization Regulators. March 1, 1983.
41. Moore, Steve, M. D. Containing Healthcare Costs Through Alternative Delivery Systems: The PPO Approach. Seminar of Healthcare Purchasors of Puget Sound. April 20, 1983.
42. Mountain Medical PPO: A Case History of Marketing a New Concept in the Denver Area. *FAH Review.* July/August 1982.
43. New California PPOs Producing Tumult Among Physicians. *American Medical News.* p. 1, 2, 9. February 25, 1983.
44. Naisbitt, John. *Megatrends.* New York: Warner Books. 1982.
45. A New Cure for Health-Cost Fever. *Business Week.* September 20, 1982.
46. O'Connor, Maureen L. Preferred Provider Organizations: A Market Approach to Healthcare Competition. *Hospital Forum.* November/December 1982.
47. Office of Technology Assessment, Medical Technology Under Proposals to Increase Competition in Healthcare. U.S. Government Printing Office. Washington, D.C. 1982.
48. Perler, J. M. Utilization Review for the PPO. *Hospital Forum.* November/December 1982.
49. PPO Hopes to "Franchise" To Hospitals Nationwide. *Modern Healthcare.* March 1983.
50. PPOs Will Proliferate If QA and UA Programs Improve. *Hospital Peer Review.* May 1982.
51. Preferred Providers: Discount Health Care. *Washington Report on Medicine and Health.* July 12, 1982.
52. Preferred Provider Organizations: A New Approach to Health Care Delivery. *Interact.* May/June 1983.
53. Rundle, Rhoda L. Little Relief in Sight for Soaring Health Premiums. *Business Insurance.* January 10, 1983.
54. Rundle, Rhoda L. No Relief From Rate Hikes; Health Plan Insurers Factor in Runaway Costs. *Business Insurance.* May 31, 1982.
55. State of the American Hospital Association, before the Senate Committee on Labor and Human Resources on Health Care Cost. May 25, 1983.
56. Stockman, David A. Premises for a Medical Marketplace: A Neo

Conservative's Vision of How to Transform the Health System. *Health Affairs.* Winter 1981.
57. Three Networks Reflect Growing Interest in the Development of California PPOs. *FAH Review.* July/August 1982.
58. Tibbitts, Samuel J. Healthcare Heads for Revolutionary Changes in Organization, Delivery. *Modern Healthcare.* July 1983.
59. White, Charles H. and Arstein-Kerslake, Cindy. PPO Activity in California Hospitals. *CHA Insight.* May 26, 1983.

Index